ORGANIZED OBSTACLES:
A COLLECTION OF WEIGHT LOSS STORIES FROM THOSE WHO LAUGHED IN IMPOSSIBLE'S FACE.
A LITERARY COLLABORATION WITH
RHONDA
-THE SUCCESS INSTIGATOR-
NAILS

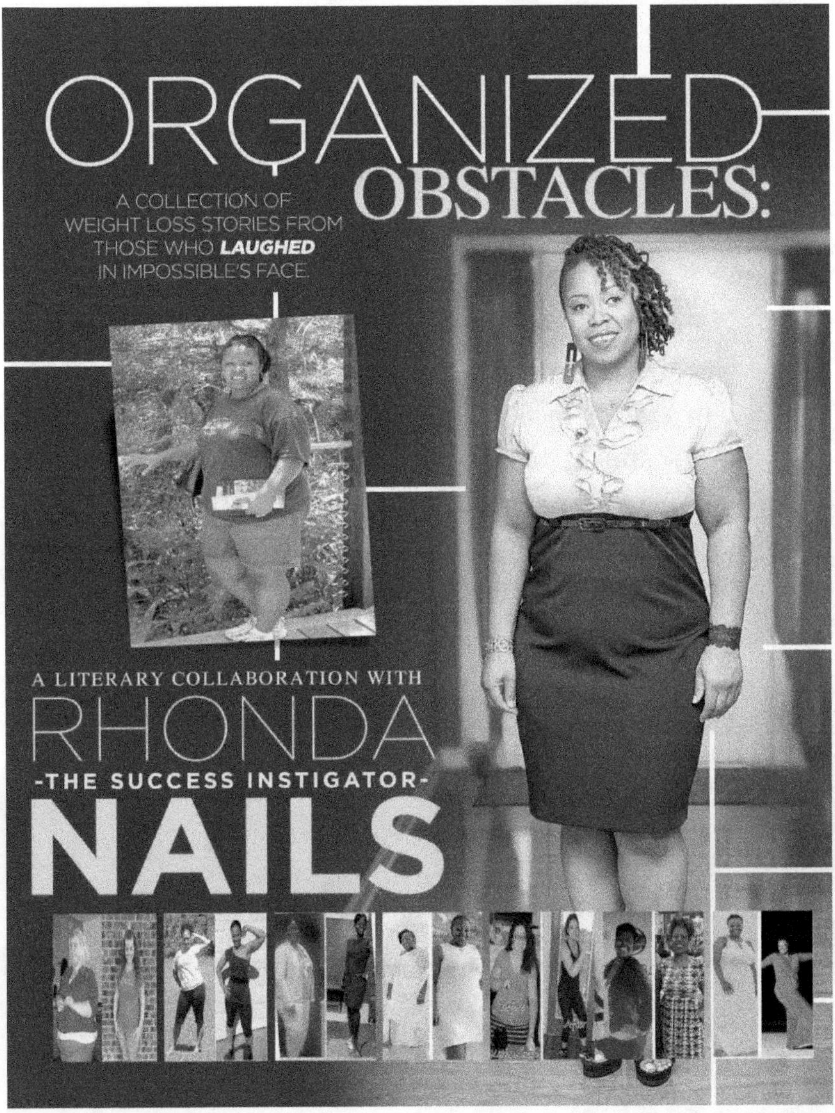

ORGANIZED OBSTACLES: A COLLECTION OF
WEIGHT LOSS STORIES

Copyright © 2016 Rhonda Nails

All rights reserved.
No part of this book may be reproduced, stored in a retrieval system, or transmitted in any form or by any means, electronic, mechanical, photocopying, recording, scanning, or otherwise, without the prior written permission of the publisher. Individual author contact information is provided within each chapter.

ISBN: 978-0-9861335-9-6

PRINTED IN USA

ORGANIZED OBSTACLES: A COLLECTION OF WEIGHT LOSS STORIES

TABLE OF CONTENTS

ACKNOWLEDGEMENTS v
INTRODUCTION vi
RHONDA NAILS' STORY 1
INSPIRATIONAL EVE'S STORY 8
MELINDA'S STORY 17
TINA C. HINES' STORY 32
KATIE KIZZIE'S STORY 44
ICY'S STORY 49
KATRINA HARRELL'S STORY: 61
CHRISTIN PEARSON'S STORY 81
MOTIVATIONAL MESSAGES 88
YUMMY RECIPES 92
ABOUT THE BOOK CREATOR 106
ABOUT THE CONTRIBUTORS 108

ORGANIZED OBSTACLES: A COLLECTION OF WEIGHT LOSS STORIES

ACKNOWLEDGEMENTS

Not everyone has two families but I do. I have my biological family that has supported every inch of my journey through thick and thin. My daughter, mother, father, and brother have been more than my support. They have been my crutches when I couldn't walk anymore. Not because they felt an obligation but simply because they wouldn't let the winner in me quit.

I also have my Fit family. These are the incredible women of P2 Fitness who were divinely orchestrated to come into my life before I was able to self-destruct. A team of Wonder Women who laugh in the face of impossibility on a daily basis and have taught me to do so not only physically, but mentally and emotionally as well.

Thank you to both of my families for wiping my tears, calling me when I didn't feel like talking, laughing with me until I cried and supported every inch of my physical journey to release the weight.

~ Rhonda

ORGANIZED OBSTACLES: A COLLECTION OF WEIGHT LOSS STORIES

INTRODUCTION

Losing weight is hard. Losing weight while dealing with major obstacles is almost impossible. Someone once said, "Losing weight is a mind game. Change your mind, change your body." This book is not about losing weight. It is about the organized obstacle that was placed in each contributor's life and how they were able to overcome and celebrate victory, one pound at a time. Every contributor in this book overcame the mental battle before they could overcome the physical one.

The 2nd book in the *Organized Obstacles* series reveals the stories of those who laughed in the face of impossibility while on their weight loss journey. More than just shedding a few pounds, true weight loss makes you examine your worth and value. We are only given one body in this lifetime. How we care for it is either painfully obvious or pleasantly appealing. This book chronicles several real life stories of those who share their weight release stories with the world. How they did it, obstacles they overcame and how they are maintaining their incredible weight release journey.

ORGANIZED OBSTACLES: A COLLECTION OF WEIGHT LOSS STORIES

I will beat her.
I will train harder.
I know her weaknesses.
I know her strengths.
I've lost to her before, but not this time.
She is going down.
I have the advantage.
I know her well.
She is the OLD ME!

-Bonnie Pfiester

RHONDA NAILS' STORY

My background

The number on the scale was close to 300 pounds . . . 270 to be exact. I was proud to be labeled a "thick chick." I had curves for days and I wasn't ashamed . . . or was I? I lied to myself over the years until the lies became my truth. The 3 lies I told myself were: 1. Big-boned women ran on my dad side of the family, 2. I was made like this and my personal favorite, 3. My man likes me with a little extra.

Truth is, I was tired of going directly to the plus size section of any clothing store I walked into. No sleeveless tops because my arms were way too big. No form fitting shirts that came above my navel because my belly poked out and I had a pouch. 2X and 3X clothing was the norm in my closet and so was the color black. I had black shirts, black pants, black capris but no black shorts. I had not worn shorts since college and my alternative was the sundress. It was easy to hide all my curves within the safety of the sun dress. No one had to know that I was pushing a size 20 because I cut the tags off all my clothes. My favorite seasons were fall and winter because I could hide my extra curves behind baggy, long sweaters and a pair of leggings. Full length pictures were out of the

ORGANIZED OBSTACLES: A COLLECTION OF WEIGHT LOSS STORIES

question. I was ashamed of all that I had gained. 10 years of shame, guilt and being overwhelmed was enough to make me want to throw in the towel. Years of feeling like I didn't have it in me was encouraged by the fact that my marriage was lifeless. Years of dealing with a spouse who didn't care, didn't encourage and didn't want change was crushing my spirit. Plus, he liked heavy women right? So losing weight would be detrimental to my marriage. At least that's what I thought and my thoughts became my reality . . . his reality. Joining a gym was not "in the budget," getting a personal trainer was too expensive, and you are fine the way you are were the lies that was constantly told by the man whom I had promised to honor 10 years ago. The battle in my mind was do I believe him or do I begin to believe myself? I was scared to change, scared that I might have to lose something. However, that is exactly what needed to happen. I needed to lose "something" in order to gain something. I wanted Rhonda back. The old Rhonda, the one that used to laugh and make others laugh, the one who saw herself as an attractive, intelligent and strong presence. That was the person I lost in the marriage, trying to appease his needs and desires, trying to be the model wife. I suppressed everything I was in order to play the role; and in the process Rhonda not only gained weight but she also gained embarrassment, shame and an overwhelming desire to give up.

I was ashamed, embarrassed and fed up.

ORGANIZED OBSTACLES: A COLLECTION OF WEIGHT LOSS STORIES

My Shift

My annual trip to the doctor changed the way I felt about myself and more importantly the image I displayed to my daughter. When I stepped on the scale it read 270 pounds. I froze. I didn't even hear the Doctor tell me to step off the scale. Instead, I was stuck in a moment of terror that I had become the person who I feared. One lonely tear fell down the right side of my face. I quickly wiped it away before the Doctor could see. As we walked toward the examination room, every step brought me closer to a grim reality. I was not just overweight, I was nearly obese.

As I sat on the examination table, the Doctor began to wrap the blood pressure belt around my arm. She stopped. Took off the cuff and replaced it with a larger cuff. My arm was too big. She stated that she replaced the cuff to get a more accurate reading but I believe we both knew that my arms were too large for the normal sized cuff. After she received the more "accurate" reading, she completed my physical exam and began to review her findings.

The first subject topic was my weight. At 5'6" and 270 pounds, I was considered at the low end of obese. My first response was going to be, "well, at least I'm on the low end." However, what came out was just pure panic. "The scale needs to be recalibrated. I'm not that heavy. I don't feel obese." These were all my excuses for not dealing with the issues I needed to face. I had hidden all

ORGANIZED OBSTACLES: A COLLECTION OF WEIGHT LOSS STORIES

my insecurities, all my shame and all my fears into my flesh. I was busy making too many withdrawals and never invested back into me. It was time to pay the piper. 12 years of fast food, lack of exercise and hiding behind spanx had come to an end.

The second subject topic was my blood pressure. Her findings were that my numbers were so high that I had no choice but to be medicated to control my blood pressure. This was embarrassing. I was only 37. Surely, no one that young should be on medication to control their blood pressure. That was for older folks. The high blood pressure readings were a direct impact of how I chose to live my life. Large contributors were my weight and unhealthy eating. Ultimately, my choices were to continue the lifestyle accompanied with medication and continued deteriorated health OR I could make a lifestyle change, get off the medication and take back my life. I'm sure you know by now which choice I made.

My Process

Typically, it takes more than 3,000 calories to make up a pound. I don't care how you weigh it, slice it, divide it or look at it. That is a lot of work! I decided that the only way to combat this issue was to do something that I had never done in order to achieve the results that I have always wanted to receive. I enrolled in a free 45 day boot camp style program hoping to kick start my weight loss journey intensely. I worked out 5-6 days a week sometimes twice a day! At the end of the 45 days, I stepped on the scale hoping to see amazing results only to find out that I had gained 5 pounds! Needless to say, I was severely disappointed and discouraged and ready to give up. My Trainer, Christin Pearson sat with me as we went over my discouraging numbers and felt every bit of my pain. She helped me gain my composure and assured me that next month's numbers would be different. Although, I wanted to believe her, my mind just wouldn't allow me to believe differently.

For the next 30 days, I got up and dragged myself to the 6AM class, planned my meals and ate as clean as I could adding a gallon of water to my regimen. I fussed and cussed but I made a deal with myself that if I didn't see some results after 30 days then this weight loss thing was history. After the 30 days, it was time to step back on the scale and get measured. To my surprise, I had lost 8 pounds and several inches! My thoughts about weight loss started to change; I thought, "Maybe I did have what it takes to lose this weight."

Over the next few months, I continued to lose several pounds and mad inches but not without the hard work and dedication to do this for me. The battle is never really the scale. The battle is how bad you want it. Do you want it at 6 am in the morning? Do you want it enough to ignore your cravings? Do you want it enough even when you don't see it working? I wanted it that bad. I wanted it for me. This was my daily gift to myself and I was not going to allow someone or things distract me from my goals.

My Life

The shift and the process of releasing the weight has been transformational. My life is so freeing now. Do I still wake up at 6a to work out?? Absolutely! Do I love it every day? Absolutely NOT! But what I do love is the gift that I give myself every time I sweat in the gym. The gift of becoming a better, healthier, stronger Rhonda. And I must say that the results in my jeans don't hurt either. I have been able to maintain this weight loss because I realized that I am worth every drop of sweat that is released from my body. Every pound that is shed is encouraged to go. I embrace my new found muscles and the way my body feels when I finish a workout.

One of the most beneficial things that I have done for myself outside of releasing the weight is change my environment. Please understand that the people you surround yourself with will be a reflection of how you see yourself. If you surround yourself with negative, manipulative and indecisive people, those are the results that you will receive. However, if you decide to surround yourself with people who continuously want you to live at your highest and best use, then that reflection will manifest. Surrounding yourself with people who encourage, support and lift you up is not an option, it is a necessity. The women and men that I now have in my life will not allow me to give up nor will they encourage mediocrity. They push me even when I don't like it. They challenge me even when I feel I am at my limit. They surround me with motivation to ensure my success.

One of my favorite quotes that keeps me going is: "The Best project you will ever work on is YOU." This time it's for me. Not for a man, not for my daughter, not for a dress size . . . simply me.

INSPIRATIONAL EVE'S STORY
From Victim to Victor

At 24 years old, I weighed 340 pounds. During an office visit with my doctor he mumbled: "If you don't make some drastic changes, you may not live to be 40," without ever making eye contact with me. He then gave me some information about diets and a dietitian's contact information. His diagnosis was startling to hear but not enough to make me want to put down the cheeseburger (the one comfort I found in life) and make a drastic change.

I hungered for more than just food. I hungered to be seen, to be heard, to be loved, to be accepted. And, ultimately, to be enough. Like Fat Bastard from *Austin Powers* said, "I'm unhappy because I eat, and I eat because I'm unhappy."

Interestingly enough, the more I weighed, the less I valued myself. The scale went up and the value for myself went down. I was bulimic and purged daily. I had sleep apnea, heart palpitations, and a cholesterol level of over 300; 200/100 blood pressure and skin problems. I loved food. I loved alcohol. I loved anything that gave me a temporary feeling of fullness, because I felt empty. I developed a lack of self-love after years of being left with empty promises and being given false senses of security. I was slowly killing myself. I was feeding an empty heart thousands of empty calories a day.

The doctor told me that my chances of making it to 30 years old could also be a challenge since I also smoked. But, that didn't scare me into action either. It wasn't until I realized I was looking into a genetic mirror that something awakened in me. At that time, my parents were ill and disabled. My mom's body was breaking down from autoimmune diseases. My dad, at only sixty-five, could no longer walk on his own. Additionally, he had congestive heart failure, small veins disease, liver failure, dementia, and hypertension.

One day after helping my dad's nurse change his diaper, I realized this was going to be my future. If I didn't make a change, what I saw before me was going to be me; a burden to myself and my family, unable to have children and not living the life I saw in my dreams. Looking at my parents, who are generally our barometer of what is possible in our lives, I felt helpless. If genetics played any part in my future, then it looked grim. I didn't want that to be me. There had to be a way to have a better quality of life. Weren't we supposed to be our parents but a smarter more evolved 2.0 version?

ORGANIZED OBSTACLES: A COLLECTION OF WEIGHT LOSS STORIES

It seemed impossible that I had the power to change anything going on in my life. There was so much swirling in every direction. The man I was engaged to was obsessed with obese women. He is what they call a 'BBW (Big Beautiful Women) Lover.' Consequently, I was obsessed with the need to be loved by a man. The very thing feeding my need for approval was the one thing leaving me empty. The emptier I felt, the more I indulged in food and substances.

And, there I was . . . 24 years young, morbidly obese, living at home with no high school diploma, engaged to a *BBW* lover; a closet bulimic, purging my overeating but not my poor life decisions. Not having much to live for, so I thought, I started contemplating suicide. It was something I journaled about but told no one. I knew people would want to talk me out of it. Why keep going? I had nothing to live for. There was nothing to look forward to other than the McRib coming back to McDonalds; there was no end in sight. I drove my mom to all her doctor's appointments and picked up her prescriptions so I had access to a large quantity of pills. I began to plan how I would do it.

One night, after eating my daily fourth meal bender at Taco Bell and confessing my savory sins to the toilet, I decided it was time to check out. I had recently found out my fiancé was in love with another woman. After throwing away the $17 worth of Taco Bell by vomiting it into the toilet and flushing it down, I caught a glimpse in the toilet water of myself. I didn't recognize her. Who was that? Who had I become? Where did my dreams go? I stood up and talked to the source of all life: God, Buddha, Universe, Spirit, and Divine - whatever you want to call it - for the first time in my life. I was done. I wasn't worth many more breaths. And in that moment, something inside me asked *"What if this time could be different?"* It almost felt like the scene in *Field of Dreams* when Kevin Costner's character hears the whisper "If you build it, he will come." I started an inner dialogue with that question for what felt like hours. Realistically it was probably only 15 minutes.

"What if this time could be different?"

I had tried the diets, the exercise programs, the fads; I would lose 60 pounds and gain 80 back. I had the talks with the doctor about gastric bypass. Nothing worked for me. Then I realized I had never tried it with a clear heart and a clear mind. *What if this time could be different?* That thought put the ball in my court to dream again. I tapped my fingers on the surface of my future as I thought about what it could look like. That seemingly tiny question took me out of being the passenger and put me into the driver's seat. *"What if this time could be different? What things could I do differently this time?"* What if I took the chance of doing it differently? What if I could actually meet the man of my dreams, become healthy, be able to have babies and rebuild the vision I once had about making a difference in the world? Maybe trying again would be worth it. But how? How would I do differently?

At this time in my life, I couldn't walk my full driveway. It was one part ability and the other part laziness. I had not conditioned myself to push past what was uncomfortable yet. So every day, from that day forward, I would throw on a men's 3X shirt, a women's 4X sweatpants, and lace up my shoes and start up my driveway. It was baby steps. This entire journey was baby steps. Once I got to the top of the driveway, I thought, "Well, how much farther can I walk?" So, my next goal was to walk my entire neighborhood. Since I was embarrassed by my appearance, I only walked in the mornings and at night. Then, when walking became easy, I would alternate walking and jogging in 10 second intervals. When I felt my exercise became easier, I would push myself a little harder. I began signing up for 5Ks. I noted the time it took to finish (the first one was over an hour and a half) and would strive for one minute better the next time.

I lost 100 pounds within 10 months because I moved daily. I drastically changed my eating habits as well. I ate on smaller plates and used smaller silverware to create the illusion I had a lot of food on my plate. I stopped eating fast and frozen foods daily and switched to eating a vegan diet. I knew I needed something that would shock my system with micronutrients and new levels of water I hadn't ever ingested. Eventually my eating changed from 100% vegan to including some meats and other sources of protein. It wasn't a diet for me, it was a lifestyle shift. I felt a greater level of pride in my life than I ever had. Cooking became one of my favorite things to do. The kitchen became my laboratory where I was able to put all of my culinary hypotheses to the test. Immersed in recipe books and ingredients, I infused everything I ate with love and creativity. Eating food was now about the designed intent: nourishment and enjoyment.

There are many ways to approach changing your diet. I found "Eating the Rainbow" helped me, in a fun and colorful way, to determine throughout the day if my body was getting the nutrients it needed. I still use this method to take note throughout my day of how much of the rainbow I eat.

Eating Your Rainbow Example:

Red: Apples, beets, red bell pepper, strawberries, tomatoes, radishes
Orange: Oranges, carrots, orange bell pepper, pumpkin, sweet potatoes
Yellow: Bananas, yellow bell pepper, golden beets, summer squash, onions
Blue/Purple: Blueberries, eggplant, purple potatoes, red onions, plums, figs
Green: Spinach, broccoli, kale, kiwis, bok choy, cucumbers, celery, zucchini

ORGANIZED OBSTACLES: A COLLECTION OF WEIGHT LOSS STORIES

This journey is exactly that - a journey. It is not a destination. I had to cross several finish lines to realize this journey isn't about the finish line. From walking my driveway to completing a half-marathon, this part of my life is about finding enjoyment in all that I do. We think that by achieving our goal weight that life will suddenly make sense. That we will suddenly approve of ourselves more. I have been able to maintain this weight loss through three things:

1. The food I eat daily and the relationship I have with it
2. Ensuring I exercise several times a week.
3. Self-Reflection.

If I had not implemented the element of self-reflection, I would not have kept the weight off. I needed to release what originally caused the weight gain or I would have easily gained it all back. There were moments I felt just how easy it would be to fall back down the rabbit hole of my former habits.

When we lose something, our unconscious mind wants to find it. When we lose our keys, our purse, our wallet or our dog, we will stop at nothing to find these things. Losing weight is no different. For this reason many people lose weight then gain it back. When you release something you are consciously letting it go. The weight loss industry treats the effect (the fat) not the cause (emotions, traumas, meanings, experiences) of why you put on the weight in the first place. I can tell you from experience, all of the insecurities and criticism you hold at the start of the journey becomes packed in your weight loss suitcase if you don't clear it out before you begin. Everything you carry on the outside is something you are carrying on the inside. Determined to never gain it back I began to understand why I gained the weight and why I wouldn't keep it off. I constantly felt like I was battling something inside me. Until I came up with my own personal strategy to overcome the weight and make it fun, I was never able to keep the weight off.

I could spend this part of my story telling you that my blood pressure has stabilized along with my cholesterol. I could discuss how I no longer stop breathing while I sleep. I could tell you stories of how I fit in one seat on an airplane and no longer need a seat belt extender. I could ramble on about how I now can shop at H&M, Forever 21 and Express for the first time in my life. Or the fact that I can tie my shoes easily, and how lovely it is to cross my legs. Yet, what has changed more than anything is how I view myself, food, and the power I hold within me.

When you climb a mountain not only is the view beautiful, but there is a better perspective of everything you just traveled over to get there. You have a sense of accomplishment when you conquer a mountain. That is how I feel. The mental, emotional and physical weight was a mountain. Conquering the mountain taught me more about myself and my own personal strength than any fat burning pill or exercise program ever could.

What no one in the weight loss industry tells you is how to handle life on the other side of the mountain or how to cope with the process of the journey. Industry experts neglect to tell you the facts about your body during this process. As a life coach and neuro-linguistic programmer (NLP), I now help learn how to release the weight once and for all. Doing this through a series of workshops and individual sessions, I am able to help others accomplish what took me five years to complete. I could not do this if I had not released the emotional baggage, mental pain and physical weight from my life.

Today, at 30 years old, I'm still alive and in the best shape of my life, I can honestly say I love myself. I wouldn't be able to say that without letting go of the former identity of who I used to be at 340 pounds. By embracing "Who I am now" I was able to let go of who I used to be.

This time was different because I chose to be different.

If you would like to start your weight release journey, visit Eve's website at www.inspirationaleve.com.

MELINDA'S STORY

My background

As far back as I can remember I have struggled with weight. Based on what family members have told me through the years, I have faint memories of being small as a child. As little girls my mother was very strict about what my sister and I ate, never allowing us to eat candy or drink sodas; until one day, the restriction was lifted. My mother no longer cared (so it appeared that way) about what we ate, and we were allowed to make our own decisions about food choices.

At ten years old, approaching middle school the pounds started coming. Nearly 200 lbs., I was larger than all my friends by the time I went to high school. Self-esteem was something I did not have because the only picture of beauty I knew was presented on television and in magazines.

When I looked in the mirror, I didn't see anything that represented society's vision of beauty. To add insult to injury, there was very little to no support from my family which set the foundation for a positive self-image. As a matter of fact, I recall being teased often by people in my own family about being fat. Additionally, the constant teasing from my classmates didn't help my self-esteem

ORGANIZED OBSTACLES: A COLLECTION OF WEIGHT LOSS STORIES

either. Names like "Bull, Jelly Roll and Pig," still ring in my head even today. My teen years were spent wanting to be accepted and loved. Believing that if I were smaller, I thought life would be different. It seemed to me that the skinny girls were more accepted and had high self-esteem. Finding safety in hiding, I spent most of my teen years in the background. During my summer vacations, I would starve myself with the hope of losing the weight. I tried only fruit diets, one meal a day routines and even started running laps around my grandparents' house hoping to run the pounds away. Nothing worked; in fact I never lost a pound.

Most summers I returned to school heavier than the prior school year. I never considered myself a heavy eater so I couldn't understand why I gained weight. My family always said "it runs in the family" so you can't help but be big; it's hereditary; was it because of genetics? Or did it have everything to do with the types of food my family ate and the lack of exercise. We ate fried foods several times a week and bread was a must for every meal. By the time I graduated from high school I weighed over 200 pounds.

I continued hiding behind the scenes and accepted that my size was just who I was and there was nothing I could do about. I believed my family's belief, which was that the weight was hereditary. When I looked around every other woman in my family was overweight. The summer after my freshman year was spent in Cape May New

ORGANIZED OBSTACLES: A COLLECTION OF WEIGHT LOSS STORIES

Jersey with one of my favorite aunts and she too had struggled with weight. Weight issues was something she and I often discussed and while spending the summer with her I was introduced to weight loss pills.

Over the course of that summer I dropped over 40 pounds and I declare to you that was the first time in my life that I began to see a glimpse of self-esteem.

That was the best summer ever; I returned to college renewed and refreshed thinking that surely the rest of the weight would disappear given how quickly I had lost the 40 pounds during the summer break. Well one can predict how that turned out. Yes, I returned with a new outlook but I didn't have the weight loss pills. So by the end of my second year I gained all the weight back and then some.

Over the next several years due to the demands of college and the death of my mother, losing weight was no longer a priority. I continued gaining weight and tried putting it out of my mind. By the time I graduated from college I approached 250 pounds with no idea of how to lose it again, so I started taking the weight loss pills again, but this program actually provided me with healthy meal options and exercise was highly recommended. This time things were different because I learned how to eat right and I exercised for the first time in my life. I dropped a significant amount of weight and was down below 200 pounds. My confidence and self-esteem came through and I felt really good about what I had accomplished. For about six months, I stayed on the weight loss pills and then began weaning myself off of them. The good thing about this part of my journey was being able to maintain the weight loss while eating healthy and exercising.

Life during this time was good professionally, spiritually and mentally.

Fast forward three years and my life took a turn for the worse. Financial problems, marriage, motherhood and unemployment caused me to experience increased stress. With this stress I stopped exercising and began incorporating old habits; along with this came the weight gain. Back up to 200 plus pounds I started trying all kinds of weight loss programs: Atkins, weight watchers, Jenny Craig, cabbage soup, black tea etc., you name it I had tried it! I lost twenty to thirty pounds here and there but would gain the weight back and then some.

My Aunt Linda was the only person, I think, who knew about my internal struggle with my weight. She was my confidant, the one person I felt comfortable discussing my struggle with. She and I had many conversations about losing weight and what life would be like if we could only defeat this battle. Of all the people I knew she was the one person that probably wanted this more than I did. Just like me, she had tried everything to lose weight without success. I'll never forget the day she called and told me she had decided to have gastric bypass surgery. I listened intently to the details about the process and the potential weight loss she could have. I heard the hope and enthusiasm in her words and her will to live. She felt like this would be life changing and lifesaving. Being one of her biggest supporters, I had a feeling deep down inside that I would follow in her footsteps. In 2006, she successfully had the surgery but due to other complications she passed away several weeks later. The pain associated with her passing is still hard to talk about today; I had lost the one person who understood my struggle first hand.

By 2008, I was divorced, dealing with the death of my father and began working a stressful job that led to more weight gain. While I was never professionally diagnosed with chronic depression, I knew without a shadow of doubt that I suffered from depression and food became a source of comfort for me. I had no idea how to cope with the stress of life. Most people, who knew me, would have never guessed because I hid it very well; often times conforming to what other people needed or wanted me to be. This was my way of gaining acceptance and hiding. Seeing myself as a complete failure, I wanted to be invisible to everyone around me. Vulnerability on my job left me feeling like I did not have a voice; having a voice meant people seeing me for who I was. Lacking confidence in myself meant being unable to convince others to have confidence in me or my work. Even with all of that, something inside told me, "If I lost the weight I could become the person I had long desired to be." Therefore, I continued my quest to lose weight, yet over the next four years I gained weight and continued the practice of hiding behind the scenes.

My shift

I remember the day that was a true turning point for me or the day I hit what I call "rock bottom." It was during a meeting with my Director and Assistant Director, in which I did not agree with what was being asked of me to do; I did not have the courage or the confidence to express my concerns. I just stood there with a lump in my throat holding back the tears, feeling like an absolute failure. This occurred prior to a meeting at my son's school. As a result of that incident; I was unable to be the advocate my son needed during that meeting . . . instead I was a pure basket case. I cried the entire time during the drive back to work, because I had not only failed myself, I had failed my son. *I had accepted living subpar and failing myself all those years, but failing my son was not an option. It was in that moment, that I made a decision to change my life and change the way I felt about myself not only for me, but for my son.* I knew that I couldn't do it alone; I began to think upon my last conversation with my aunt and the hope she had for life with her decision to have the gastric bypass surgery. Prior to that moment I had never given the decision a lot of thought. I always associated her passing with that surgery, but on that day the idea and decision was clear.

ORGANIZED OBSTACLES: A COLLECTION OF WEIGHT LOSS STORIES

I contacted Duke Metabolic Weight Loss Center that day and began the process that would change my life forever. Everything went extremely smooth to my surprise. I heard how intense the process was and had prepared myself for stumbling blocks along the way; yet for me not one road block presented itself. My doctor said I was the perfect candidate because I had no preexisting conditions, my vitals were in good shape and nothing indicated that there would be issues post op. My doctor was more concerned about my family history of cancer, high blood pressure/ hypertension and diabetes; I was reminded that if I continued to carry the weight around, I would be at high risk of developing one or more of the diseases that had invaded the lives of so many of my family members.

I hadn't shared with my family the decision to have the surgery because I didn't want anyone to talk me out of it; quite honestly it was something I had to do for myself.

I had completed all the steps to qualify and the next step was to receive a surgery date. Several months had gone by and I hadn't heard any communications from Duke regarding my surgery date and I began to think that it wasn't going to happen. I started a weight loss program with my family that consisted of weekly weigh-ins and individual commitments to live a healthy lifestyle by eating better and implementing exercise into our daily routine. I was completely caught off guard when I received the call from Duke that would change my life

ORGANIZED OBSTACLES: A COLLECTION OF WEIGHT LOSS STORIES

forever. The nurse on the other end of the line was talking about a surgery date and pre-op procedures and I was on the other end speechless. She called my name at least three times before I could speak and when I spoke I know my words came as a surprise to her. I said, "Ma'am I don't know if I can do it." There was silence on the phone for a few seconds and she finally said, "Ma'am you've completed the process and the next step is to bring you in to perform the procedure." I said, "I understand that but I'm nervous and don't know if I can go through with it." She said she understood and would leave the surgery date scheduled for September 11, 2012. Additionally, I needed to call 24 hours in advance of pre-op if I wanted to cancel the surgery.

I went home that evening and I prayed all night for an answer from God. My entire life had flashed before me during that moment of seeking direction. Memories of an unhappy childhood, abuse and bad relationships that resulted in years of low self-esteem, lack of confidence and lack of self-love; to me those were the reasons why I continued to pack on weight through the years.

When I woke up the next morning everything was clear and God had given me direction. I knew without a shadow of doubt that this would be the tool needed to rid myself of the pounds in order to get to the true issues which had me at such a dark place for so many years. On 9/11/12, with my family by my side, I underwent the gastric bypass surgery. The day of surgery I weighed 261

ORGANIZED OBSTACLES: A COLLECTION OF WEIGHT LOSS STORIES

pounds and I made a commitment to myself that I would give 100% and become the best version of myself that I could be. Surgery went extremely well, and I knew right away that I had made the best decision of my life. I had been afforded a tool that would allow me the ability to reach my weight loss goals for once in my life.

My process

The afternoon following surgery, I requested assistance with getting out of bed to walk around the hospital floor because I was determined to keep moving and not be idle. Everyone was surprised that I was moving around so quickly and encouraged me to take things slow to allow proper healing. I admit . . . I was weak but I was so eager to give that 100% I had committed to.

The procedure had been done and now it was time to do my part. There are so many people who undergo weight loss surgery with the notion that "I'll lose the weight no matter what" while never incorporating healthy eating or exercise into their daily routines. I was and am still determined, today, not to be part of the statistics of patients who gain the weight back. Upon release from the hospital, I was on a liquid diet for two weeks which consisted of protein shakes, broth, sugar free jello and water. This was the hardest part of the process, and the only time I had questioned my decision. By week two, I began to regain my strength and was walking around my neighborhood 10 mins at the top of every hour. By week six, I began a soft diet which consisted of foods such as soft meats, vegetables, eggs and soups. I walked 2 to 3 miles a day and lost over forty pounds.

Once released from my doctor's care, I implemented running into my walking program. Running was something I had enjoyed doing but due to the weight I was unable to run long distances. I'm thankful I learned early in the process that exercise would be the key to my success.

Although, I dropped pounds due to the weight loss surgery, I knew the day would come that my body would stabilize. For me, that day came rather quickly. Most gastric bypass patients are only able to consume a small amount of food during one meal; after six months this was no longer the case for me. I was able to consume amounts that were not typical and my appetite had increased significantly. My doctor attributed the increase in appetite to an increased metabolism rate due to running. While I ate small portions every two hours, I found myself hungry all the time. I ate three meals a day including two or more snacks. Being a creature of habit, my meal options were pretty consistent. This made grocery shopping and meal preparation very easy. When shopping for food, I only shopped the perimeter of the grocery story focusing only on fresh foods like fruits, vegetables, dairy, meats and fish. My breakfast almost always consisted of two slices of bacon (turkey or pork), one scrambled egg and one piece of toast. For mid-morning snack, I always chose some type of fruit. My

ORGANIZED OBSTACLES: A COLLECTION OF WEIGHT LOSS STORIES

lunch included meat and vegetables with a starch included occasionally. My mid afternoon snack was generally a protein shake or nuts. For dinner, I mainly focused on vegetables and some source of protein. Before bed, I would always end the day with a snack such as plain, Greek yogurt with fresh fruit or sugar free pudding. As you can see my diet was jammed pack with lots of calories which is the fuel needed to keep our metabolisms functioning properly while generating the energy our bodies need. I think it's important to mention during my weight loss process that I never eliminated anything from my diet. If I craved something, I allowed myself to have it; of course, within moderation (never over indulging). I would have it but make adjustments in other areas. Adjustments included things like increased exercise, low calorie food options for other meals. Honestly, my diet was pretty boring but it worked for me. The moment I had to think about it too much or spend hours planning for a meal decreased the likelihood of me sticking with it.

Running was my sole source of exercise, something I'd always had a passion for and knew that If I ever loss the weight, I would take it to another level. I never missed a scheduled run. I ran through the rain, heat and bitter cold; I was determined that nothing would stand in my way. The more I ran the more my body craved it; I couldn't get enough of it. Four months after surgery, I completed my first organized 5k in fewer than 45 minutes. My body changed right in front of my eyes; I lost weight and inches. Every week my endurance was getting better and I was able to run faster and longer distances. I was running at a rate that I never imagined myself being able to. I started competing in more organized races and set a goal to compete in a ½ marathon in honor of my one year anniversary. In order to stay motivated and prepare for the ½ marathon, I participated in many 5ks, 10ks and 10 milers. In fact, I not only participated in organized races, I stood out in ways unimaginable. I competed in the Great Human Race and came in 5th place for my age group. I was featured in Endurance Magazine for participating in the Tar Heel ten milers. One year later, I had reached my weight loss goal and had lost a total of 110 pounds and the following month completed my first half marathon in honor of my one year anniversary. I ran the entire race without stopping not even for water, and not one time did I get tired so I knew the training had paid off. As I approached the finish line, I could hear the crowd cheering and chanting things like "You're almost there," "Way to go," You're Awesome" and "Great Job." It was in that moment that I believed I am truly awesome.

Maintenance

This year, I will celebrate my four year anniversary since I had the gastric bypass surgery and I have been able to maintain my weight within 10 lbs. give or take. I attribute my ability to maintain my weight to running. On average, I still run 20 – 25 miles per week as part of my fitness regimen. I always try to get in the recommended daily water amount and practice portion control during my meals. Eating every 2 – 3 hours has allowed me to control cravings and impulse eating. I've developed a daily regimen where fitness is a priority and working out is the first thing on my daily list of activities. Making sure I keep my annual follow up appointments with my bariatric surgeon has been a very important factor in meeting and maintaining my weight loss goals. These regular visits ensure that my body is functioning properly and processing food in a manner that it should be. The best advice that my surgeon gave me prior to surgery was that this process should be treated as a tool in order to meet your weight loss goals and nothing else. Heeding to the doctor's advice has enabled me to remain successful thus far on this journey.

My life

My life has changed in so many positive ways since losing the weight. My whole being has been impacted. I'm better physically, mentally and spiritually. Prior to the weight loss, I admit, I was spiraling out of control and was at a poor physical state of being. Things are much clearer now; and I can now see to the surface and understand the underlining issues which created the weight gain. Understanding and recognizing root problems is the first step toward correcting any problem. The most profound and revealing part of this process had nothing to do with food, but everything to do with the

ORGANIZED OBSTACLES: A COLLECTION OF WEIGHT LOSS STORIES

unresolved issues from my past. While most of the issues are still there, I no longer suppress them. The weight loss has given me the courage and strength to face them head on. I'm a better mother for my son, setting positive examples of a healthy lifestyle. We do fun fitness activities and prepare healthy meals together. I've inspired my immediate family to start running; completing 5ks with my older sister and two nieces. On an annual basis I participate in Carolina Godiva Running start program as a pacer, assisting beginning runners; teaching them how to run. This is a program I participated in many years ago when I first learned to run. I've had so many people contact me to tell me how I've inspired them to lose weight or reach their fitness goals. I'm always so humble and touched because never in a million years did I believe I would inspire others to reach their fitness goals.

From the very beginning of my weight loss process, I shared my weight loss journey via social media in hopes of inspiring others to reach their weight loss goals. I knew that would be my biggest avenue to reach people who are struggling with weight issues. In addition to sharing my story via Facebook, I created an online fitness accountability group which allows people to share their fitness goals and accomplishments. This group is inspiring, encouraging and uplifting. I can always count on the members to encourage me when I need it the most! When I look back over my weight loss journey, there is nothing that I would do differently. It hasn't been an easy process but it's been worth it. Every day is a day of recommitment and dedication and some days are better than others but I can honestly say that since September 2012, the good days have outweighed the bad days. I give all glory and praise to my Lord and Savior, Jesus Christ. I'm grateful for this opportunity to share my story, because I know that there are many people living behind the scene trying not to be seen just as I was. I hope my story will inspire someone to stop letting others define who they are and take the steps necessary to release the baggage in order to become the person that they desire to be.

ORGANIZED OBSTACLES: A COLLECTION OF WEIGHT LOSS STORIES

TINA C. HINES' STORY

When you suffer from depression, you never know the impact it will have on other areas of your life. For instance – for me, it was weight gain that was triggered by a prescription I needed to help alleviate my depression. Although one of the side effects listed on the pharmaceutical literature was weight loss, it somehow had the opposite effect on me. My weight soared to 193 pounds, and it didn't take long for the excess weight to become more than I could bear on my small frame. After seeing a picture of myself, I realized that something had to change. I had to make a lifestyle transformation!

In order for you to understand my journey, I need to dig deep to revisit where it all began. I never would have imagined that one phone call in December would send me into a tailspin of emotions that ended in clinical depression. The phone call was from a woman telling me that I needed to travel to Georgia immediately because my mom had suffered a ruptured cerebral aneurysm and had been rushed to the hospital. I was in shock and felt numb. Unsure what to do first, I rushed home from the office, started calling my mom's siblings, and then prepared to travel to Savannah, Georgia.

ORGANIZED OBSTACLES: A COLLECTION OF WEIGHT LOSS STORIES

The next morning I arrived in Georgia, where I would stay for longer than I had envisioned. Seeing my mother in the hospital heavily sedated with a tube that looked like a pipe extending from her brain was a terribly emotional experience for me. For days she endured tests while I held vigil at the hospital conversing with doctors, specialists and nurses to ensure that my mom would receive the best care that would ultimately lead to her recovery.

Within weeks, my mom was transferred to a rehabilitation center for physical therapy to continue her healing. She was eventually released from the hospital a few days before New Year's Day. Once she was comfortably back in her home and resources were put in place for her care during my absence, I prepared for my return to New Jersey, a place that was my sacred space of peace.

How Did I End Up Here . . . Suffering from Depression? Depression, or any mental health condition, can be a challenge and is often considered a silent health issue – silent because it unveils itself so quietly that the person who is suffering often does not realize that there is something changing within. That is exactly what happened to me.

When I returned home from Georgia, something felt different. I walked into my home, greeted my son, and placed my suitcase at the foot of my bed where it stayed unopened for a period of time. I climbed into my bed and thought, "all I want to do is stay here." I was physically and mentally exhausted. During the entire time that I was caring for my mom, whenever I was sleeping, I was not really resting. After replaying the Georgia experience in my mind, I discovered that, in the midst of my mother's storm, I forgot to take care of me. Physically I was perfectly fine, or so I thought, but mentally I was drained.

Over the next few days it became more and more difficult to get out of bed. I like to say my bed would not release me. However, I did manage to get up and go into the office every day. But the struggle remained, and there were times when I just wanted to crawl under my desk and cry. I couldn't understand why I was feeling like my body was failing me. With a great deal of apprehension, I decided it was time to call in the experts to help me figure out what was going on with my body and find something – anything that would help me get back to the woman I was before I boarded that flight to Georgia.

Off to the doctors I went and after observation and conversation, my physician informed me that I was clinically depressed. My first reaction was denial because I don't get depressed. I handle everything with a smile and always view life from a positive perspective. However, considering I had never experienced depression before, of course denial would be the first reaction. Denial quickly shifted to acceptance as I thought about the old saying, "The first step to recovery is admitting you have a problem." I had a problem and I wanted it gone because I was not feeling like Tina.

Now that I had accepted that I was clinically depressed, it was time to put into action the necessary steps to start the healing process. I began practicing daily meditation to reconnect with the woman within and honor all that I was experiencing; I attended weekly therapy sessions with a licensed clinical social worker to discuss my emotional highs and lows; and with much trepidation I accepted the prescription meds. My motto was that I could work through it, whatever IT was. Unfortunately, although my mouth said that I could work my way out of these new emotions, my mind and body were telling me that I could not. The latter prevailed because I did not have enough fight in me. All I could do was listen to what my body was telling me. It was telling me that I needed to practice self-care.

Over time I was prescribed a variety of medicines to help with my clinical depression. However, I soon discovered that although the medicine eased my depressed symptoms, it was having an adverse reaction on my weight. It appeared that every time I visited the doctor for a check-up my weight had increased by 5 pounds. At this point I mentioned my weight concern to my doctor. She too was amazed, because in the past patients would lose weight. Eventually she placed me on a medicine that did not impact my weight. By this time my weight had increased to 193 pounds.

I was concerned about the increase in my weight but unable to focus on my mental health and physical health at the same time. It was too overwhelming for me at the time. That is until I caught a glimpse of myself in a picture that nudged me to take action. This image is one forever etched in my mind.

What's In a Picture?

There is an English idiom that states, "A picture is worth a thousand words." A picture that was taken the spring of 2015 spoke to me and that was when I made the decision to take my health serious. Reflecting on my visits to the doctor for checkups and noticing the increase of the numbers on the scale all started to hit me like a ton of bricks. It had not totally registered in my brain that I was buying clothes in larger sizes and that I needed to do something about my weight until I saw that picture of me wearing a white dress.

It was the final day of my yearly retreat in Anguilla, and my clients and I were having a photoshoot on the beach. I was smiling, striking model poses and feeling very cute. The photoshoot captured images that would eventually be used for marketing my coaching business. Yet once I received the final images and looked at the picture intently, I saw the puffiness of my face, the tired look in my eyes, and the overall unhealthy condition of my body. The images revealed what had been happening on the inside of my body months before. I often share a quote, "When you feel good internally, it is exuded externally. No make-up required." Viewing those images of me revealed that I was not feeling good on the inside as it pertained to my weight. That photo was the first incentive for me to start reducing my weight. The other incentive was walking through my closet that contained clothes ranging from a size 4 to size 18.

The interesting thing about this revelation was that I was coaching a client on the very thing I needed help with personally. I was guiding her towards identifying the blockages that caused her weight gain. Meanwhile, she was also working reducing her weight by making a lifestyle change that included the use of weight loss products.

I must be perfectly honest, I am not one who enjoys exercise. I don't like to sweat and the gym and I are not friends. I tried it. It was not for me and I moved on. Many people laugh at me when I say that I am allergic to the gym. But that's 100% Tina. Perhaps you are wondering, if I did not exercise, what exactly I did to lose over 30 pounds?

A client who attended the retreat in Anguilla shared the program she was following to lose weight. I was not new to trying weight loss products. Therefore, I asked several questions in order to make an informed decision. Based on our conversation and from what I had observed during our sessions and retreat, I made the decision to give it a try. In my opinion, it beats not trying at all and staying stuck and uncomfortable in the same place with the same weight.

Time to Make a Lifestyle Change

Losing weight involves more than exercising or using nutritional supplements to support you on a weight loss journey. It should also include an overall lifestyle change. I had finally accepted the fact that a lifestyle change is what I needed!

Everyone who decides to lose weight must do what works for them in order to achieve the desired results. When you apply what works for you, you are less likely to give up. What worked for me was using nutritional products from Total Life Changes (TLC). TLC provides superior nutritional supplements, skincare and weight loss products designed to aid in transforming your health. The products I specifically used included resolution drops (which suppresses the appetite and burns fat); Iaso Detox Tea (which cleanses the impurities from your system without harsh stimulants); and last but not least, the NutraBurst liquid multivitamin. These three products, coupled with a low calorie meal plan, were the main products that helped me lose over 30 lbs. Perhaps

ORGANIZED OBSTACLES: A COLLECTION OF WEIGHT LOSS STORIES

you are wondering how this is possible with little to no exercise. Very simple . . . dedication! I was dedicated to the process of losing weight. I was dedicated to looking and feeling healthy. I was dedicated to me.

As a reminder, I did not exercise. Allow me to elaborate in order for you to understand how this is possible. First I increased my daily water intake. I dislike water but understand the importance of hydrating my body and flushing my system. The instructions for the resolution drops included a food list to follow during its use, which meant I had to reduce the intake of carbohydrates like bread, rice, pasta, sweetened beverages and just about anything that contained sugar. The one item that I refrained from eating for 6 months was rice. That was actually easy. However, the toughest part of this regimen was avoiding bread. I love bread, especially hot bread. I have little to no willpower when it comes to bread. However, I did have a little help in that department.

Every once in a while my son and I would dine at the Olive Garden. If you have ever dined there, then you are familiar with their warm breadsticks. On one occasion I instructed the waiter to place the basket of breadsticks near my son. By placing them closer to my son, I would be less inclined to eat one. That lasted a short time because eventually I asked my son to give me a piece of bread. He gave me a stare somewhat similar to the one I would give him when he was in trouble, and then he said, "Mom??" We debated back and forth until he gave me a

ORGANIZED OBSTACLES: A COLLECTION OF WEIGHT LOSS STORIES

piece of bread. All I could do was laugh, and you would too if you saw the size of the piece he gave me. I was literally unable to even taste the bread. All I could say was, "Seriously??" His response was so cute that I was unable to say anything else thereafter. He said, "Mom, you are doing so well. You don't need that bread."

Another way that I avoid eating bread is through visualization. Imagine the process of making bread. Flour, yeast, water and whatever else are key ingredients in creating dough. Then the dough is allowed to rise for a number of hours before being placed in the oven to bake. Now, close your eyes and imagine eating a piece of bread followed by drinking a glass of water. That bread is rising in your stomach in the same manner. Not a pretty vision but it was an effective one when bread was calling and I wanted to resist the temptation.

My eating choices soon changed, and I began to incorporate more fruits and vegetables along with lean cuts of meat and fish. There was a time when bacon, egg, and cheese on a bagel would be my breakfast. With my new found love for my *Nutribullet*, every morning I created a green smoothie with strawberries, bananas, kiwi, and spinach. My smoothie keeps me full until lunch and also is a great replacement when I have a sugar craving or want ice cream. When I say that weight loss is possible by paying attention to what works for you, I actually mean it and have achieved the results to prove it.

ORGANIZED OBSTACLES: A COLLECTION OF WEIGHT LOSS STORIES

During my weight loss journey, a funny experience took place when I was meeting with a client in New York. She and I were seated on a couch having a discussion. I stood up to write notes on the whiteboard, and my size 12 jeans were sliding off my waist. She and I laughed as I exclaimed, "I think I have a problem and it's a good problem. These jeans are too big." Later that evening, I went through my closet and started gathering jeans that ranged from size 4 to 18. After trying them on, it was clear that some were too small and others were too big. I decided it was time to end the relationship with the smaller and larger jeans that were no longer my size.

I have decluttered my closet of the clothes that no longer fit. What remains are those that I like and fit as they once did. Now when I feel the need to go shopping for clothes, I simply venture to my closet and pull out my old new clothes because they fit. They look great on me, and I feel great wearing them. That's what it is all about – looking and feeling great about yourself.

The Secret Is Out and a New World Opened

Here is the big secret to weight loss, at least for me. Once you know the culprit (problem) of your weight gain, you will discover what needs to be done (solution) in order to transform your weight. My culprit was not food or depression, it was medication. Once the medication was changed, I no longer gained weight. However, I did not lose weight either. This meant that I needed to figure out

ORGANIZED OBSTACLES: A COLLECTION OF WEIGHT LOSS STORIES

what was making the excess weight stay on my small frame. I wrote down everything, and I mean everything, that I consumed. Then I decided what was important to me – those foods or my health. My health won and I started to remove unhealthy food from my diet or consumed them in moderation. Considering I am the one who purchased the groceries in my home, the solution to my problem was not as hard as I initially thought it would be. It was just adjusting my mindset and staying dedicated to my health.

There is always a lesson to be learned in life. At the time when class is in session we may not fully understand the lesson and its purpose. However, eventually it will be revealed. The weight loss journey was a road I needed to travel in order to rediscover Tina. This journey reminded me that it is essential to practice self-care of my mind, body, and spirit. When one of these components is not in alignment, eventually the others will falter. The key is detecting it early in order to tackle the issue.

In the past it was hard for me to embrace the weight I had lost because I shed a lot of weight in a very short period of time. Whenever I would look at myself in the mirror I was amazed and at the same time perplexed. Mentally it had not fully registered that I was smaller than I had been in years. During this weight loss journey, I chose to lose the weight at a slower pace. I was in no rush. All I wanted to was to look and feel healthy. I was ready physically and mentally for what was happening to my body. As the weight started coming off, I celebrated every five pound milestone that got me closer to my goal.

Now that the weight is finally off and staying off, I have been able to share authentically the highs and lows of this weight loss journey. I am honest about using the Total Life Changes products and my decision to make a lifestyle change. I was not working on a beach body, summer body or whatever many choose to call it. I was working on my everyday body to improve my health to look and feel good according to Tina. I feel healthier than I have felt in years. I owe it all to my decision to make a lifestyle change.

ORGANIZED OBSTACLES: A COLLECTION OF WEIGHT LOSS STORIES

KATIE KIZZIE'S STORY

In the summer of 2014, I was a tired and overweight 34-year-old mother of two. I had never consistently exercised and I hardly paid attention to the foods that I was eating. I had reached my heaviest weight during my first pregnancy seven years prior, at a weight of just over 215 pounds. I was ashamed then, but not because of my appearance. Instead, because I couldn't easily walk up the stairs and found myself unable to catch my breath moving from one level of my home to another. I chose to blame my exhaustion on the pregnancy rather than my lack of exercise and poor nutrition. During my second pregnancy, I was diagnosed with gestational diabetes and the diet I followed to manage my diabetes also served to help manage my weight. But once I delivered my son and the diabetes disappeared, so did my dedication to eating better. And the weight I lost after that pregnancy came back just as quickly as all the pounds before.

Like many women, I always admired others for their dedication to living a fit and healthy lifestyle. I had hoped the same for myself, yet I could never get organized ~~to get there~~ on my own. Never having been an athlete, and not growing up in a home with a focus on physical fitness, I slogged through whenever I did get the chance to work out. My personal drive wasn't there; I had given up and resigned myself to being out of shape. I hated summer and dreaded having to sweat it out in capris or jeans while it seemed like everyone around me was far more comfortable in their skirts and shorts.

With two young children, I rarely had the time to focus on anything other than the needs of my family. For years, I heard myself say to my husband, "I just want to be healthier, for them (our kids) and for me." I wanted to lose weight so I could run after them and play the games they begged me to, like all the other parents. We would join other families at a local park for a cookout, but I felt too ashamed to play kickball because of the extra weight that slowed me down and asthma leaving me breathless with the slightest exertion. I was tired of making excuses...

I discovered a local boot camp gym focused on women; they were running a special – 45-days free, with no commitment at the end of the term. I thought, "Why not? There's no financial commitment and I can get some guidance on how to quickly lose a little weight for free." I truly had no idea what I was in for . . . The boot camp workouts were HARD, to say the least; yet the guidance and training met me where I was, not where I wanted to be.

Even with exercise, my nutritional choices have been my greatest struggle. I find the most success when I track my macros – focusing on maintaining the right ratio of protein, fat, and carbohydrates each day for my body. My

ORGANIZED OBSTACLES: A COLLECTION OF WEIGHT LOSS STORIES

carbohydrate intake is my weak point. Having grown up in North Carolina, my grandmothers loved me through food; they instilled in me a tremendous love of a nice warm biscuit slathered with butter and homemade preserves.

I do best when I plan my meals ahead of time. If I put the time in on Sunday, then my meals for the week are all ready to go. When I crave sweets, I find almonds to be a great substitution, especially the cocoa-dusted variety. The easiest habit for me to break was my soda addiction. Drinking only water has helped me drop quite a few pounds and shave plenty of inches from my waistline.

Over the past two years, with consistent workouts and nutritional guidance, I have dropped over 30 pounds – from 184 to 152 – and moved from a size 14 to a size 8. But more importantly to me, I have completed a 5-mile-run and can chest press my 8-year-old daughter (to her great delight). At the end of April 2016, I am proud to say that I completed a 10000-rep week of workouts – which means that, over the course of 4 days, I finished 10000 reps of exercises that worked my upper body, core, lower body, and endurance. I finished every workout absolutely exhausted – and I have never felt better in my life!

It's been almost two years since I decided that I was worth the risk. I risked my pride and my time to see if I could lose just a little weight. Before, I preferred to sleep as late as possible on a Saturday morning and my idea of a good workout was fifteen minutes on an elliptical machine. I never could have imagined I would be running laps voluntarily, doing burpees at 5:00 AM, or going all out for 45 minutes (or more) in a row with minimal breaks. With the right support and an awesome fitness program, I have made a lifestyle change that has me on the road to reaching my dream goals.

My desire is to work out five to six days a week, which isn't always easy. Recently, some health struggles kept me from making it consistently; some weeks I missed the gym altogether. The struggle to get back into the swing of things hasn't been easy, but I'm doing what I can to get back to where I was before. I find that the more often I go, the better that I feel both physically and mentally. Keeping a consistent schedule helps me immensely – whether working out in the mornings or in the evenings, if I am there each day at the same time, then my body adjusts to the schedule and the expectation that I will return the following day at the same time.

Today, I love that I never come into the same workout two days in a row. Constantly pushing my body out of the comfort zone and going harder than I believed I was capable of, I exceed the limits once holding me back. The consistency found in my personal trainer (Christin Pearson) has been the foundation for my lifestyle change and she has inspired me to do better for myself. I believe in myself again and have discovered a desire to work as hard as I need to in order to reach my full potential.

ORGANIZED OBSTACLES: A COLLECTION OF WEIGHT LOSS STORIES

The best part of my lifestyle change has been the increased energy that I have each day! I can play outside with my kids . . . running around and roughhousing at the local park without feeling overwhelmed or overexerted. I can go for a run without instantly needing to reach for my inhaler after 5 minutes. Coworkers and family members have commented on how inspiring my change has been for them; continuing on this road to my fittest self with hopes to lead more people toward making lifestyle changes and finding their fitter selves is my goal. I am truly most thankful for the positive impact that my healthier lifestyle has had on my kids' choices – seeing my daughter eat healthier meals and exercise more because of the choices she sees her mom making on a daily basis is amazing.

ICY'S STORY

Journal entry April 21, 2011 4:44 am

As much as I didn't want to, I need to do this. I need to write! I don't know if there is a book, play or sitcom in this or if it is just for me, but I'm compelled to write this now! I was watching OWN's "Addicted To Food" and I see myself in most of the people on this show. I am Tinisha, in the documentary who is embraced in the fat. The fat was "my lover," it seduces me, it comforted and protected me like a man does a woman, or so I thought. Was it because mommy didn't hug and kiss me or daddy didn't tell me he loved me or that I was beautiful? Did it make me unattractive so men wouldn't want to feel me up while my family slept like my cousin did when I was 12? Did it allow me to make many stupid decisions about my choices in lovers, and toxic relationships and friendships? Now that I am older, wiser and still struggle with "my lover," I fight not to ever go back to that place that makes me so tired and feel so ugly. I have been so busy or making excuses like I'm too busy to work out, that once again I put my appointment with my personal trainer and my therapist on hold! Once again I put me on hold, why? Do I love me? Why do I sabotage myself! I think about food. I never did that before the surgery . . . it's bothering me. I can't go back to "my lover." He is not good for me. He smothers *me, holds me back and makes me feel so ugly! But I'm walking out of the forest, into an open clear path, where I can see things a whole lot clearer now. Thank God! Watch out world, I hope you are ready for me! Here we go......*

As I look back on my life and I look at myself, I often wonder why I never became a drug addict, alcoholic or a prostitute? There were many moments when I was between the ages of 11-14 years old, I thought about killing myself. I just didn't feel beautiful, because of the words I grew up hearing. I remember my paternal grandmother, Elsie, would always say, "you're soooo pretty, if you could just lose some weight!" What the hell did that mean? Am I ugly because I'm fat? I can't be fat and pretty at the same time? Those words really messed me up mentally, made me really angry, defensive, scared and ashamed.

These words from Elsie, along with words from many other people who claim to love me, set off a chain of events in my life that could have killed me.

One day I remember thinking of slitting my wrists because I found out that William, the cutest boy in my class whom I had a crush on, didn't feel the same way about me. In the cafeteria one day I heard these kids laughing and pointing at me; I overheard him talking about how fat I am and how he could never like an elephant like me . . . wow! Just two nights before we sat on the phone and he told me how pretty I am and what a good friend he thought I was! "Why are people so cruel God?" He was always so nice to me one on one, but became very nasty when he was with his friends . . . this hurt my heart. Going into the bathroom, I remember crying my eyes out; not understanding what I did to deserve this treatment. I couldn't wait to get home, so I didn't have to see these people that I thought were my friends.

One afternoon sitting in homeroom waiting for school to be dismissed, William attempted to talk to me. Looking at the clock I thought, "three minutes is not up yet? Where's the damn dismissal bell, I'm dying here!" Sitting by myself on the bus, I cried while staring out the window. Phony friends asked, "Why are you crying?" With no reply, I simply waited for my stop so I could get away from it all.

When I reached home, my mom was cooking dinner; I said good afternoon and went straight to the bathroom, with my books, to hide. The bathroom was a favorite place . . . why? I don't know. There was a pink fluffy rug that I would sit on and write in my dairy, or just go to cry. That day I went there to think how I could end it all. "*Maybe I should drink this Tylenol, daddy has razors . . .*" That seemed to be the in thing with the white kids back then.

I just sat on the floor and cried and started to pray: "*God, it's me, can you hear me? Can you help me? Can you save*

ORGANIZED OBSTACLES: A COLLECTION OF WEIGHT LOSS STORIES

me? Can you make the pain in my heart stop? Does dying hurt? Why don't you answer me? Pastor Sessoms said suicide is a sin . . . is that true? I don't wanna go to hell, but I can't go back to school again. Can you hear me GOD?"

Rocking back and forth I started humming *His Eye Is On The Sparrow*. My grandmother taught me that song to sing as my first solo; to this day the song brings comfort to my soul. My humming became loud singing coming from the bathroom 'til my tears began to dry up and I heard my mother yell "Icilma! What are you doing in that bathroom? Come eat your food gal!" That is when I knew God was watching over my life. Listening to the words in the song I began feeling a sense of calm over my heart. Starting to feel like I would be ok, I thought, "my mom and my sisters would need me . . . I can't kill myself, well at least not today."

Walking out of that bathroom, I still felt a little hurt, yet looking at myself differently. Not as the elephant William said I was, but beauty in my God's eyes. Being the oldest, I spent my life as the protector, leader, and example for my sisters; not being someone else in my mother's life that would fail her. Wanting people to be proud of me, I strived to do well in school, to be the first college graduate, not to be a teen mom, not be on drugs; just so people would see more than my weight. However, I have one question, who was the example for me? Who was the leader for me? Who protected me from my

ORGANIZED OBSTACLES: A COLLECTION OF WEIGHT LOSS STORIES

cousin England, who would climb in my bed and sexually molest me?

Allowing men to use my body sexually for what I thought was love to comfort me, who protected me then?

Looking at my obese body, I realized that every pound represented a layer of protection . . . a layer of armor from the life that I was living. Food became my protector. Food has always been a part of my life in good times as well as bad. Someone died . . . we ate; happy times . . . we ate. That was all I ever knew. You would think at this point I would hate it.

I remember going to visit the nutritionist once a month with my mom, because I was 14 years old and almost hitting 200 pounds . . . What shame I felt about that. I remember how nasty the Nutritionist was to my mom about blaming my parents for why I was so fat! I think that is why I became a Nutritionist years later, because I never wanted another child to feel the way I did that day in the Nutritionist's office . . . like a failure.

As I became older the effect of food on the body intrigued me; I wanted to know why I looked the way I do and why when I ate something, my body changed for worse and not better. It's a shame that when I should be happy being a teen, I'm obsessed with calories and my weight. This led to years and years of yoyo fad dieting, over the counter and medically prescribed diet

ORGANIZED OBSTACLES: A COLLECTION OF WEIGHT LOSS STORIES

medication which almost drove me to a state of depression.

As mentioned earlier, I decided to study Dietetics, Food and Nutrition in college in an effort to "save myself" from this fat suit I had created around me. As I progressed in school I realized that the food represented so much more than food for me. Food allowed me to bury the past hurts in my life, it allowed me to "put off" facing what the real problem in my life was.

I never addressed being molested as a child, never told my parents, and never faced the person who had hurt me.

My poor behavior went on for years. I carried those bad habits into my adulthood; burying my problems with food and not addressing my feelings. As a result of my love for food, I ate myself to an unhealthy weight of 407 lbs. This became a turning point for me, as I thought I was going insane. Seeking the help of a mental health therapist, I needed advice regarding gastric bypass surgery. Clinically, I knew the surgery was a temporary Band-Aid and I needed to finally address the underlying issues of guilt, depression, molestation, the abortion and other factors affecting my weight gain crisis. My therapist helped me greatly in these areas, digging deep into my pain.

I had the surgery, lost 165 lbs. and kept the weight off about five years. Life happened. An accident causing me to require knee and shoulder surgery, steroid treatments to my spine left me depressed. This depression led to me gaining 75 lbs. My 'lover' had returned. Yet, this time, something was different within me.

Social media connected me to a Life Transformation Specialist by the name of Tina C. Hines. I began to follow her posts and subscribed to her monthly newsletter "Sister Friends." Through attending one of Tina's workshops I was able to begin a journey of healing within. As mentioned, my therapist helped me, however, with Tina's help I was able to find forgiveness within myself. Concepts such as self-love became real to me and began to overcome past decisions leading to guilt, shame and sabotage.

Tina helped me release the pain through journal writing. Through her teaching, I learned affirmation writing and writing my destiny on paper. Meditation became a key source for healing my past wounds. Visualization helped me see my smaller, healthier body being strong and full of energy. My personal and professional relationship with Tina flourished as she continued helping me take my life back through her teaching. Loving me began to take place; love, self-confidence and change glowed through me. Tina shared with me about her annual Caribbean retreat, "Remember Me;" and I told her I would be there. As the retreat was months away, I continued working on my emotional wounds and weight loss journey.

ORGANIZED OBSTACLES: A COLLECTION OF WEIGHT LOSS STORIES

Scrolling through social media one day, I came across some photos posted by a good friend. With each new photo, she looked smaller, therefore, I reached out to her in hopes to find out what she was doing. She introduced me to a weight loss company and product, Total Life Changes (TLC). She advised that she was using the detox tea and that the products were all natural. Her testimony consisted of her doctor removing a lot of medications she was taking, lowered blood levels and toxins beings released from her body in addition to losing weight. As a dietician, I was curious about this product and thought, 'I've tried every diet and weight loss medication known to man; trying this would not hurt."

Being a carbohydrate addict, white flour and sugar are not my friends. They love my hips and thighs. Detoxification was crucial for the weight to come off so I began to let go of breads, pasta, potatoes, and rice . . . the fire starters as I call them. The weight started falling off. During this process, journaling was important for me as well. Writing affirmations about my new body helped me visualize the smaller dress I would be able to wear while riding the plane to the retreat.

In addition to journaling, taking pictures of my progress helped me remain focused; I kept it to myself, at first, and did not even share with Tina.

My energy increased; so I was able to take long walks, one to three miles at a time and felt good about it. My friends saw a chance in me, Tina did as well. In one of

ORGANIZED OBSTACLES: A COLLECTION OF WEIGHT LOSS STORIES

our sessions she asked me what I was doing because she could see the emotional, spiritual AND physical transformation taking place in my life. Finally, I had given myself permission to love myself and change my eating habits. Tina was proud of my focus and progress. This time I was in a place of pure self-love and self-care.

While on the retreat, Tina asked all attendees to write a letter of things we wanted to release. Releasing what no longer served me allowed me to make room for the blessings I wanted in my life. Writing a "Dear John Letter" to my 'lover', the unwanted weight, I began by saying "Goodbye." In the letter, I have myself permission to release 'him.' He, the weight, held me back from opportunities, made me question my self-worth, and weighed my spirit down. Continuing, I told my 'lover' that our season had come to an end and he was no longer welcome in my life. Additionally, I thanked 'him' for the life lessons but advised I am stronger and the new found love I have for myself was all I needed, so he could go. Tying the note to a balloon I released it into the Anguillan sky. Standing there on that white sandy beach I watched until I could no longer see the balloon and I cried tears of joy because releasing the balloon representing my emotional weight as well as the physical. I felt the release of my child hood pain; the silly decisions which I had made in the past . . . the guilt, shame flew away with that balloon. Renewal occurred in my

ORGANIZED OBSTACLES: A COLLECTION OF WEIGHT LOSS STORIES

body . . . I felt free. The next day I left Anguilla ready to begin the next phase of my weight journey . . . to be back at home with a new and improved mindset

When I returned home, I took more pictures of my feet on the scale as my weight continued to go down. This is when I decided to share my journey on social media and become transparent about what I had gone through. By sharing my journey, I believed it would be a blessing for someone else. Additionally this would provide accountability for me, as well as be a therapeutic way for me to stay focused. By sharing, I was able to create a weight loss community and online support system for others. This online community gives me a sense of purpose, allows me to mentor other women and provides me the opportunity to help others who feel as though they are alone in this journey.

In addition, I created a workshop called "One Moment For Me," in which I teach women about taking a moment to practice self-love and self-care; affirmation writing and meditation are also key concepts taught in the workshop. As a result, I have become certified as a Reiki Practitioner and Holistic Life Style Coach. These certifications along with my nutrition degree, my healthier mindset and knowledge of using therapeutic grade essential oils empower me even more. Total Life Changes had been a significant part of this journey, therefore, I became a distributor. Within the past year, I was promoted to Executive Director in the company.

ORGANIZED OBSTACLES: A COLLECTION OF WEIGHT LOSS STORIES

To date, I have lost 75 lbs.; since I left the beaches of Anguilla. Tina C. Hines provided me with a lot of tools which guided me and I have taken those tools implemented them for myself and now teach them to women all over the world.

Life will always happen yet I am well armed to fight off carb cravings by eating more leafy green vegetables, drinking water and avoiding white flour, sugar, fried foods and by using TLC detox products. This is what I did to lose 75 lbs. Although I lost more than that years ago, this new weight loss is much more significant for me. This is different because I no longer worry about the number on the scale; I celebrate because I can sit in the airplane seat with the armrest down. My bracelet falls off my wrist now; I was able to donate my bigger clothing, my size 22 skinny jeans are looser now and I am ready for size 20 . . . this is why I celebrate. My knee is healed since 2014; I could only walk for 15 minutes and in 2015 I was able only able to walk one to three miles . . . but NOW I can walk four to five miles without collapsing . . . that my friend is progress!

ORGANIZED OBSTACLES: A COLLECTION OF WEIGHT LOSS STORIES

ORGANIZED OBSTACLES: A COLLECTION OF WEIGHT LOSS STORIES

KATRINA HARRELL'S STORY:
Drastic Weight Loss

*"As above, so below, **as within, so without**, as the universe, so the soul. . ."*
Hermes Trismegistus

Drastic Weight Loss Tip #1 - Courage to Change

"I love you"

The eye burn began. Tears began to slowly yet steadily form in my eyes as I repeated those words silently over and over again . . . not to anyone, but to myself.

Staring into the bathroom mirror of my two bedroom townhome, I shared with my two children 6 and 10 and my then partner of 12 years, my body, 340 lbs., summoned up the courage to look itself in the eyes and repeat those words - directed at me; in hopes it would reach a yet unfounded depth of my soul.

"I love you, Katrina."

ORGANIZED OBSTACLES: A COLLECTION OF WEIGHT LOSS STORIES

I've said *"I love you"* many times before. I tell my children daily how much I love them. I told my partner, even my parents and my friends. Those three words are repeated by me so often that even a stranger or new acquaintance would receive what I hope are the warmth and sincerity with the sound of those words. The words "Love liberates" were tattooed on my right wrist after hearing Maya Angelou express the greatest purpose of love - to courageously free a person, allowing them to soar and become the highest version of themselves.

How ironic, looking at my body, with its increasing pains, unexpected limitations and heart palpitations, sleep apnea, irritability, and moodiness - I didn't feel like the highest version of myself. I felt - trapped.

Even being 188 lbs. overweight, I have loved myself and thought highly of myself. Yet I had never . . . ever, at 35 years old looked myself in the eyes and turned those words on me. The meaning of self-love extended beyond the mere *appearance* of love, this time; the type of self-love that ensures you're well kept, groomed or respected by people . . . the type of self-love that says we are to accept ourselves no matter the circumstances or physical condition.

The kind of self-love that is more about self-preservation than actual liberation.

ORGANIZED OBSTACLES: A COLLECTION OF WEIGHT LOSS STORIES

The kind of self-love which doesn't truly challenge the depths of your soul nor require you to fully accept the fullness of your potential; because to do so would mean the only option you have is to change. . . courageously, everything you know yourself to be which isn't connected to your highest purpose.

The self-preservation type of self-love is about creating safety on what *has* become, what is already seen - instead of what is becoming - the unseen. Inside surgery.

That sort of love in action is superficial to the type of love I found myself confronting.

The courage to come face to face with the challenge of actually being IN LOVE with myself -the unseen of what *is* my own becoming.

Loving Versus Being in Love

The emotions I felt crying in the mirror repeating the words "I love you Katrina" were the type of emotions which typically have no words. These emotions were similar to expressing the depth of love you have for your own children. It is was as if I had discovered something that was always there that I hadn't paid any attention to. Somehow, I had gotten by for 34 years simply loving myself and I thought that was enough. Successful by most accounts, despite a challenging childhood, I had managed through faith, family, drive, perseverance and

ORGANIZED OBSTACLES: A COLLECTION OF WEIGHT LOSS STORIES

determination to avoid many childhood challenges growing up that would have easily made me a negative statistic.

I knew how to stand up for myself, not allow people to take advantage of me, avoided "bad boys," finished school, worked in prestigious companies and even became an entrepreneur. I was confident and loved myself, truly.

Loving myself became more an act of obligation than true deep relationship after a while. When you're in love with yourself it's more than just the act of loving which many people who don't love themselves are capable of doing. Mostly out of an obligation to preserve oneself. Being IN love is about curiosity, appreciation, exploration, understanding, compassion, constant forgiveness. It is an understanding of the evolution of oneself. It's more of an experience that influences specific acts of love. It's the complete liberation of fear that you're contained to only one version of yourself - Limited and bound to your history, past, story, fears.

Being in love is appreciating what you've been through but recognizing it serves you no longer as there is a deeper more profound experience yet to be discovered.

For me, it's always wanting to know what else I can do for me, what else I can heal.

ORGANIZED OBSTACLES: A COLLECTION OF WEIGHT LOSS STORIES

I decided that moment, tears streaming fully down my face that I was going to find the courage to accept I needed change. I didn't know what that would actually look like; I didn't know this time what the weight loss steps would look like. I had tried every weight loss program so I knew the "steps to losing weight." This time I wasn't seeking that. I was seeking relationship with myself. To break free from a shell of acceptable living.

How does this relate to weight loss? In every possible way.

I've never in 35 years, confronted the depth of the love I have for myself. I've never seen how genuine and sincere I am. I've never allowed myself to witness the impact of my own love directly pointedly specifically on me.

It is something magical about looking into someone's eyes. Try looking into your own.

It's powerful.

I saw me . . . Katrina, a version who was trying to breakaway but couldn't. Trying to be seen and heard but had lost the tuning of her own voice. I knew how to act in self-love, but never how to BE in love with self.

Seeing my own eyes - the harsh reality of what I had deprived myself of - startled me.

ORGANIZED OBSTACLES: A COLLECTION OF WEIGHT LOSS STORIES

I never hated me, but I wanted to change. At 340 pounds, I didn't know what exactly needed to change.

But now, this was different. Because I couldn't lose the weight, not literally. I could lose the weight, but then I would find it, put it back on and yes . . . add more. This time, at my absolute heaviest, I had the reality punch that this wasn't about just losing physical weight. It was about change and courage and confrontation. I knew it, I sensed it and felt it. I just didn't know where to start.

I didn't just want to be slim again, I wanted something more. I wanted to be in love with Katrina.

Whatever courage I had to muster up it would need to be drastic and deep. Having plenty of practice as a strategist . . . knowing how real change happens in an organization and business, I knew I had to get to the root of the matter and dig deep.

Just the THOUGHT of making a drastic change in our lives sends many of us into a whirlwind of "what ifs" and anxiety of how disturbed our lives will be once we make the change. Change is scary. The thought of change is scary and that fear paralyzes you.

But I knew something had to be done because I felt trapped.

Still looking in the mirror I cried; I felt and saw my eyes swell with tears, I wanted.to hide my face but I had remembered watching a video about the ability for strangers to fall in love simply from looking into each other's eyes for 4 minutes. So I kept staring. I wanted to see if that effect would happen to me.

I never made it to four minutes. After about 30 seconds I was bawling. Uncontrollably I was sobbing in my hands as if I was trying to hide my face from judging onlookers who may have thought I lost it. Except, there was no one looking at me - except me. What had happened to me? Not just physically, but emotionally, mentally? Who was I? What was I doing here? Here in this body, here in this home? Here in this world?

I loved me, but I didn't recognize me anymore.

I didn't recognize my soul anymore.

Drastic Weight Loss Tip #2:

"You look like what you've been through. " - TD Jakes

To understand how to lose weight you have to be aware of the journey that got you there to begin with.

As if it were never going to change, I had to learn to love my obese body; and I don't mean deciding to dress it up in spanx and form fitting stylish clothes and call myself "curvy." While I love the idea of appreciating your body for its own inherent worth regardless of its size - our

ORGANIZED OBSTACLES: A COLLECTION OF WEIGHT LOSS STORIES

bodies can do marvelous things - I don't however subscribe to the idea of dressing up what one isn't willing to confront if that thing is harming you. My body, while curvy and shapely, was slowly killing me. I had sleep apnea, waking up at nights with headaches and a tight chest; I didn't have my menstrual cycles and often had pelvic pain. My knees were always in pain and my left hip would sometimes just give out; not to mention the mood swings, tension and anxiety I developed as a result of feeling so out of control. I could stand on stages speaking to audiences teaching self-love, spirituality, motivation and business, but I was slowly dying. Despite that, I first decided I had to love my larger body through true compassion for myself; realizing that whatever got me here I had to let go of; making peace with it so I could truly heal.

As mentioned above, understanding how to lose weight means you have to be aware of the journey that got you there to begin with. You look like what you've been through. The weight- or anything you struggle with - is a result of what you have been going through. It's the outcome, the result of some neglect or circumstance. It's never about food. It's always about what food does for you. Just like any other vice - food or inactivity becomes a source.

For me, food wasn't a source as much as it was a way to connect to myself - it is for most people, even those who are at a healthy weight. Food is a way we connect, but for me, it became my primary way as I began to lose myself in my own life.

After having children, a series of jobs I hated and just settling into a busy life, I stopped doing the things I enjoyed like Martial Arts, regular working out, long walks, reading, writing songs, quiet time alone. All the things which made me "me" and connected to my Source. That discontentment sneakily came upon me in form of settling into a warm bowl of peach cobbler, or the extra helping of chicken parm but no exercise (because life is too busy)!

It replaced my emotional connectors from before. Before when I was triggered, I'd go walk or work out or write, now when I became triggered, I did nothing, cried, or was complacent.

I stopped choosing my joy.

Learning to love my body parts was a challenge but I did it first. I knew if I could confront my larger than life thighs, my stomach that drooped over and touched my thighs then perhaps I could begin to reconnect with my joy.

That first day looking in the mirror became more days of looking in the mirror. First saying I love you to then pointing out body parts I loved. My skin was smooth, my shape was still beautiful to me. I recalled things I used to

ORGANIZED OBSTACLES: A COLLECTION OF WEIGHT LOSS STORIES

do that I loved; things that soothed my heart when I felt sad about something. Changing nothing else about my diet, I did this work for weeks and weeks.

Sitting quietly after putting the kids to bed, I began reading a lot more. This led to telling the truth about my own happiness in my relationship, my business, my role as a mother . . . just everything.

When I came out of the emotional spot I was spiritually freed - spiritual weight began to drop. That old part of me – which was the weight died. In that space I was born and made new. Eventually my decisions changed and I stopped doing things, unrelated to food, which I once did. Suddenly doing these things just didn't make sense for me. As my emotional and spiritual life strengthened, my physical choices changed and I cut out all beverages besides water or unsweetened tea. I stopped drinking milk, instead I challenged myself by drinking almond milk. Additionally, I researched food to gain an understanding of how it impacted my mood.

For me I did not want to be slim for the sake of being slim. I wanted freedom, liberation; a better understanding of my path and journey. Believing in and becoming the product of the spiritual teachings I heard growing up is what I wanted; instead of falling into the gap of contradiction which says we should have an abundant life but suffer in pursuit of it. Understanding my purpose, without complication and what it meant to

ORGANIZED OBSTACLES: A COLLECTION OF WEIGHT LOSS STORIES

live an abundant life seemed simple and that is what I wanted.

In the past, I tried all sorts of diet plans – from Weight Watchers, LA Weight Loss, to The Paleo Diet – you name it, I tried it. By the time I began college, I had trimmed down to a curvy 155 lbs., though I was a chubby kid and fat teenager. In college, I loved fitness and maintained a healthy weight by eating balanced meals and working hard. My display of self-love was one that many felt inspired by. Yet now I had become the result of years of neglect, emotional baggage and spiritual contradictions.

This time around I let my spirit lead and in doing so it had me on a path of self-discovery, drastically burning away any and everything that never or no longer served me.

Drastic Weight Loss Tip #3:
"... but how do you want to feel?"

Those words rang in my head like a gentle yet unrelenting bell similar to a grandma looking you in your eyes sincerely lovingly yet unflinching. I heard the words of my dear friend and coach Akilah Richards.

"Katrina... but how do you want to feel?"

The country, and soon to be world, knows her as Radical Self Expressionist coach, writer, author and "Unschooling

ORGANIZED OBSTACLES: A COLLECTION OF WEIGHT LOSS STORIES

Expert," yet I knew her as friend, sister and my own personal spiritual liberator.

We've had many video conference calls, she in Atlanta or Jamaica and me in North Carolina, some mutual strategy sessions; two newly discovered friends enjoying time. We had purposed coaching sessions where I allowed her "in" to see my soul and realize it wasn't recognizable to me- fully; it was weighty, heavy, and I was carrying so much.

I had become hidden behind expectations, pain, rejection, responsibility, dogma and fear.

I didn't know me anymore it seemed.

Relationships, parental and romantic mostly, did more to affirm what I wasn't than what I could be. Carrying everyone's pain, I made myself responsible because I knew I had the capacity in my heart to love. My soul became heavy, and so did my body because I allowed people's pain to be the focus of my love, rather that the focus being on me.

I neglected my soul and followed my body. Everyone became more important to me than me.

While I made my new choices and decisions, I focused more and more on how I felt and how I wanted to feel. This sounds so simple but it's not. Often more than not, we ignore our feelings as we are often told that our feelings and emotions can't be trusted. That is true to an extent but we have emotions and feelings for a reason. Our feelings help us pay attention to what is or isn't working. Our feelings also capture our attention and sort of say "hey, so what's going on here?" Without feelings we wouldn't know our passions or even know if we're following our calling.

It's those feelings of joy, happiness and contentment we think is a result of something happening on the outside of us. Yet in reality it's a feeling we get to conjure up anytime we want. We get to decide on the feeling we WANT and pursue the things that bring about those exact feelings. There are entire books and practices on this very idea and I am a student of how this works.

Every single day, while I made simple food choices, I decided on food choices, based on not how I FELT as that wouldn't always lead to the best choice for me, but on how I WANTED to feel.

I've always loved fruit, but in the past if I wanted to be comforted, I'd eat some sugary or starchy food. However, fruit gave me the same satisfaction as the starchy sugary foods without any of the side effects of feeling bloated, jittery, or sluggish. I had to choose my feelings; and be a freaking watch guard over them. Once I got that "feel good" feeling after eating a bowl of perfectly sweet grapes and still having energy to play with my kids, I wanted that feeling more and more.

Eventually, how I WANTED to feel was all I pursued. Journaling every day I began writing more about what made me feel content and happy. What were the real dreams and visions I had for myself? All the things that had become a stressor for me I began reimagining myself fully enjoying and the resulting feelings. Every choice or decision and feeling led me to discovering more courage. Confronting things within myself, I had to denounce what wasn't really serving me. Once I realized that my feelings and desires were 100% within my control I was led to make bolder and more courageous decisions which had nothing to do with my physical weight; rather they had more to do with my purpose and vision or learning to be in love with myself.

I never STOPPED loving food. In fact, I became more obsessed with food, cooking it, preparing meals, experimenting and of course devouring it. I made peace with my emotions and the fact that I love food. I accepted that YES I love food . . . but it is not my Source.

"How do you want to feel? Do you feel like you truly have a choice and option in how you live your life or do you feel you are simply trying to "get by?"

Drastic Weight Loss Tip #4:
   "What do you see when you see?"

ORGANIZED OBSTACLES: A COLLECTION OF WEIGHT LOSS STORIES

Vision.

For many this very well could be step one, yet in my case it wasn't until a little later that I began focusing on a new vision for my life. It wasn't until I confronted my weight and had the reality of needing a reason to shed it once and for all that I realized I needed a clearer perspective of my calling in life. Avoiding truly looking at me also meant I avoided seeing into me and thus the full scope and depth of the higher calling Creator had for my life.

You can never BE what you can't see. You can never GO where you don't know exist.

My thoughts: *"I've always known I had a purpose, I was living it . . . somewhat. I was a college graduate with bright ideas, ambition and determination. I was motivating to others. I started innovative businesses, helped peers realize their business and life dreams and was often sought as a catalyst and strategist. I had a solid relationship, I had the lifestyle on paper I always dreamed of having. I worked from home, my partner cared for us and I was an entrepreneurs and self-employed. I wrote books, spoke to audiences."*

But it didn't feel right. So what did I do?

I stopped my work . . . closed my business . . . wrote a book, and embarked on a spiritual journey to discover more of my calling. By this time, I was down 50+ lbs., I was walking or exercising everyday no matter what. My diet was enjoyable. I didn't feel tempted by food anymore. I was having fun exploring my calling and my world and subsequently food that I didn't mind if donuts were brought into the house. Before I would be so mad that my partner would bring home donuts knowing I was trying to lose weight. I used to think he was sabotaging me. This go round I become completely unbothered by it.

I was eating mindfully, playing around with vegan and vegetarian diets. I discovered that certain foods didn't respond well to my body and made it more challenging for me to release weight.

Drastic Weight Loss Tip #5:
   "As within so without . . ."

As aforementioned, my inner world changed. I started looking in the mirror at my body and began pointing out the things I loved. I started to pray and visualize my body - as my own body - but able to do things I wasn't doing, such as running or kickboxing, which I loved in college.

I wasn't having regular periods and I still had sleep apnea but I didn't focus on that. I started reading and watching videos, articles and books on metaphysics, Bruce Lipton who talks about the minds capacity to heal our own bodies.

ORGANIZED OBSTACLES: A COLLECTION OF WEIGHT LOSS STORIES

Visualization forced me to stay as present with it as I could. I stopped comparing my body to someone else's body as I'd often did. I started looking at clothes again, putting on make-up, sprucing up my outfits as best I could.

I made a decision that I was going to let go of negative ideals about what other people thought of me. I thought I had to reject food and push away from the table . . . but I didn't. I LOVE food. I made peace with it

I started drinking water first.

Then walking.

I'd walk my kids to school and pick them up.
I decided not to drink my calories because I love food. I simply changed my strategy. I'm a strategist and had be used to teaching others how to literally make any idea work for them by getting to the root of their business problems. So I turned that on to myself and my relationship with my body. I loved food. I loved cooking, loved veggies. I took things slow.

Within 2 weeks, the sleep apnea was gone; the knee pains were gone and the *cramping* ended. Within 2 weeks of that I had my period and every month after that my cycle regulated and became normal.

ORGANIZED OBSTACLES: A COLLECTION OF WEIGHT LOSS STORIES

". . . but how do you want to feel?"

The better I felt, the more I studied, the more I prayed and focused on staying present the more I got clear about my purpose in life the more I stayed consistent. Before long I didn't crave sugars or bread anymore. In fact I can't stand juice as much anymore and if I do eat a sandwich I peel most of the bread off or request gluten free or high grain versions.

I pay attention to how food makes me feel. Certain foods make me sluggish and when I'm sluggish I can't focus on my work. Which I love or time with my kids which I love.

Purpose makes the difference. If you have no clue why you're here, where you're going or nothing to drive you, changing is impossible. But with purpose nothing is impossible because that change becomes a necessary part of the journey.

Drastic Weight Loss Tip #6:
". . . You were never meant to carry the mountain but to climb it."

My weight release is slow but noticeably steady. I have released over 100 lbs. over the past two years. My lifestyle is all about increasing my self-love barometer - expanding it; this means I don't diet. Instead I focus on ways to love me by paying attention to how foods make me feel. Foods that don't make me feel light and energized or motivated I don't eat – or I eat rarely because I made a promise to myself to feel good. Feeling good is my priority, therefore, I deny myself nothing. Now, I pay attention to how my body responds after I eat something or how I feel.

Purpose ... purpose ... purpose; why I am really here. I ask, "What do I really want for me and my children? What is that nonnegotiable contract I have with my God, myself and my purpose?"

I'm 105 lbs. down as of the compiling and release of this book. I have 50 more to go for my own ideal weight. Usually I don't weigh myself; only about once every three months or more and I only do it at a nutrition center where I get more information than JUST the scale size. I have slow months where nothing happens. I stop trying to count how much weight I'll lost in a month because of my life I'm releasing and building in so many areas weight is just a part of the overall process. There is no bad or good food unless the food is synthetic. If it came from the earth it's all good; it's just in how we process it.

I have a loving relationship with food. I speak to my food, I enjoy a burger if I really crave it and I've seen my body respond accordingly. I do not deprive myself and my body takes care of the rest

ORGANIZED OBSTACLES: A COLLECTION OF WEIGHT LOSS STORIES

Drastic Weight Loss Tip #7:
 "Love Liberates"

I wanted liberation. True liberation. To be free from any mental or emotional strongholds that kept me trapped. My life is blessed, not that I don't have troubles, but troubles don't have me. I understand how God is positioning me. As a result, I follow only my truth.

ORGANIZED OBSTACLES: A COLLECTION OF WEIGHT LOSS STORIES

CHRISTIN PEARSON'S STORY

Life before working out...

Before I began my weight loss journey I was heavy and I didn't even know what working out and going to a gym was like. I had just graduated with a BS in education and unfortunately at that time no one was hiring for any teaching positions. I had gained weight during college, gained weight in an unhealthy relationship, and gained weight being stressed; felt like my life had come to an end. Being the biggest one in my family and amongst my friends, I was HIGHLY self-conscious about the way I looked, the way I felt, and the way my clothes fit.

Despite what the temperature was outside, I wore BIG HOODIES OR SWEATSHIRTS all the time. My entire life felt like it was falling apart and I felt horrible about myself, inside and out; feelings of jealousy, self-comparing consumed me and I always wished or hoped I did not look the way that I did.

Next stop... finding a job.

Of all places, I started working at a gym at the front desk. With this I received a free membership; I had no clue as to what I was doing, or where to begin. This huge place was full of elliptical machines, treadmills, stair masters, dumbbells, barbells, and other machines... what was I to do? Where was I to start? Of course I did what most new gym members do, and that is start on the treadmill doing no other than . . . you guessed it . . . walk!

You show up to this place with all this fancy equipment and all these people that seem to be experts and you don't want to look ridiculous, so you walk.

A few trainers at the gym taught me how to use the equipment and put together workouts; I began to work out with them. Doing those exercises I remember feeling like a complete failure and feeling silly for lifting such lightweight; I felt like my body was too big for what they were trying to get me to do. Feelings of weakness overwhelmed me; I felt fat and preposterous. "Why did I have to do all of this in order to get this weight off," I thought. "This should not be this difficult." Feeling as though everyone in the gym was judging me from head to toe and like no matter how hard I tried, how well I ate or how hard I worked out the weight was not going to come off I told myself, "maybe I was meant to be big forever . . . maybe I wasn't meant to lose weight. This was too hard!" "Do I quit? Do I keep going?" I asked myself.

After time, patience, consistency, dedication, and motivation I FINALLY started to see progress . . . I slowly but surely overcame my social anxieties within the gym and started to focus on what was important. . . ME! At this time my unhealthy relationship had come to an end, I came to terms that teaching was not in my forecast so I tried figuring out what was next career wise for me . . . I was ready for a physical, emotional, and mental change. My health was the only thing I could control. Who would have thought I was in control of my own health? If I could control nothing else, I thought, "at least I would look good." This first time around I lost 27 lbs. Then I met the man who is now my husband. As a result of him taking me out to eat daily, buying desserts and more, I gained the "happy weight." Additionally, I became mommy, overnight, to his two beautiful girls causing me to lose all the 'me' time I had worked desperately to find.

Gaining all the weight I had lost with a few extra pounds for fun, I had to refocus and refine what I wanted my body to look like, how I wanted to feel when I saw myself in the mirror and how I wanted to see myself in pictures. After refocusing my mind and getting back on track, I lost 30 lbs. Down to 144 lbs., which is the second go round, I was so happy to see the progress being made and the direction I was moving in. On my way to being the smallest I had been in many years, I was excited and then guess what? I found out I was pregnant . . . and not only was I pregnant I was 12 weeks, 3 days 'preggers' and *missed* my whole first trimester.

The pregnancy was beautiful . . . I gave birth to a baby boy and named him Micah. When Micah was five months old, I found out I was pregnant *again* (yes you read that correctly). Fifteen months after giving birth to my first son, I gave birth to another beautiful baby boy,

ORGANIZED OBSTACLES: A COLLECTION OF WEIGHT LOSS STORIES

Nehemiah. With the first pregnancy I gained 54 lbs. and with the second I gained 23 lbs.

After having two babies in less than two years, I was at my heaviest. As a result, I lost my muscle gains; my bod fat had sky rocketed, my self-esteem plummeted and my bod image was practically non-existent . . . I was worse than when I started my first round of weight loss.

At this time I transitioned to being a trainer; I had found my career path. This is what I loved to do and was blessed to be able to do it on a daily basis; helping women not to feel the way I felt. Now I was helping them overcome any and all negativity they felt about themselves. This time was different; my body had changed in so many ways, thanks to my beautiful bundles of joy. My body was different. This time I had 'relearned' myself and what would work vs. what would not . . . I had to start over, *again*.

This time was different because I had eyes on me . . . all of these strong, beautiful and amazingly unique women stood in front of me while I trained them – *me* . . . 183 lbs. of fat . . . no muscle. They watched me *every day*. It was important for me to not only talk the talk but also walk the walk. Not making excuses, I got my mind right. I did not make excuses. I did not let my 16 month old son nor my 6 week old son become an excuse, neither did I let them hold me back from my personal goals – husband, full time job, four children, three dogs and a house to take care of – but that did not hold me back.

ORGANIZED OBSTACLES: A COLLECTION OF WEIGHT LOSS STORIES

Additionally, there were all the women who counted on me to be there for them; amid them sending me texts, emails, or phone calls . . . I still found time for me.

THIS TIME . . . I was determined that it would be my last time around. I worked hard, DAILY, sometimes 2 to 3 times a day.

While on this journey you not only have to work out but also eat right. The hard part is not just in the gym; most importantly it is in the kitchen. Changing what you eat is hard and it does not happen overnight. Losing 50 lbs., I was the smallest I had been since I was fourteen or fifteen years old – from a size 14/16 to a 4/6. Watching myself lose the weight was positively incredible; clothes that were once a struggle to get into were now falling off of me. The person I had become, I loved. I loved helping, watching and being a part of so many other women's journey, as they got closer to their goals one workout at a time. This time . . . I reached a point of thankfulness, gratefulness and was beyond blessed to have found what I was meant to do in life.

By staying dedicated, motivated and determined I have been able to maintain my weight loss and move further into my journey. Everything about my life has improved. Determined to keep me on the list, I am healthier by far and able to keep up with my children. The list, you know the one that so many of us have yet we don't have US on it. We have everyone and everything else on it, but we always forget to add ourselves. By being determined to

ORGANIZED OBSTACLES: A COLLECTION OF WEIGHT LOSS STORIES

keep sight of how important I am, I am able to help guide my children on the right path – a healthier, happier life; and I am able to be happy for my family, taking care of them. Although I am the healthiest and happiest I have ever been, I do enjoy a cheat meal . . . I do not eat the right things 24/7 . . . I splurge now and then . . . I have not cut ALL the fat, sugar, sweets or other unhealthiness out of my life . . . yet I have learned to control what goes in my mouth. Minimizing my portions, not eating out all of the time, and being mindful of what I buy are things I practice – making smart choices for me and my family are what's most important, not being on a 'fast,' diet, or eating like a rabbit for the rest of my life.

This is a lifestyle change, not only for you but for your family. Teaching the next generation how to fuel their bodies with food, maintaining a healthy life which in turn leads to a healthy mind, body and soul is what it is about. Being able to help change the lives of many women and men is an amazing position I am blessed to be in. Watching women grow, change and achieve goals they never thought possible is awesome – watching them laugh in the face of Impossible. Thanks to my journey I get the pleasure of doing what I love on a daily basis; I get to see women who watch their whole lives change as they gain self-confidence while losing body fat, pounds, inches and seeing their clothes fit differently. It is a pleasure for me to see their bodies change; their arms, legs and core take definition. We have such an amazing group of "Fit

ORGANIZED OBSTACLES: A COLLECTION OF WEIGHT LOSS STORIES

Fam" at P² Fitness and I am blessed to be surrounded by them.

ORGANIZED OBSTACLES: A COLLECTION OF WEIGHT LOSS STORIES

MOTIVATIONAL MESSAGES

Don't let anyone derail your destiny, trip up your trajectory or f$%k up your focus!
Connected Woman Magazine
www.connectedwomanmag.com

Live healthy, Be healthy, Do healthy, is a great path to Lifestyle changes.
FitQuest For Health, LLC
http://fitquestforhealth.com

"You deserve more than some 'me time' you deserve a 'me time' routine. You hear all the time that you have to make time for yourself, that's all well and good but truth is we are all busy. I used to be the woman who figured the busier I was the more productive I was. Instead, I was left broke, sad and exhausted. To become self-care aware is not about your weekly mani/pedi it's beyond that. My self-care awareness movement is about calming the storm within us, not around us by setting boundaries and creating a daily self-care ritual that help you make yourself a priority so that you can be a better you.
I Am Self-Care Aware
www.iamselfcareaware.com

ORGANIZED OBSTACLES: A COLLECTION OF WEIGHT LOSS STORIES

The body does not understand opinion." What this means is that, no matter what we prefer in taste or texture, our bodies cannot process all that we choose to ingest. We have to feed our bodies what it needs. Too many of us don't realize that we are malnutritioned. We don't have to look like big bellied children for this to ring true. Now, not all of us are the same. So one size does not fit all. We must take the time to feel our way through what our bodies need.
The Health Conscious Diva
www.natashapennant.com

1. You're not what you consume but a byproduct of what is eating on you.

2. Losing weight is a journey and not a sprint to the finish line.

3. Being overweight isn't the problem, freeing yourself from the weight of complacency is.

4. Shedding pounds is 10 percent physical and 90 percent mental, emotional, and spiritual.

5. When you learn to lose the war against people's perception of you, the internal battle is already won.

6. Counting calories minus a healthy lifestyle, will eventually put your life in the negative.

ORGANIZED OBSTACLES: A COLLECTION OF WEIGHT LOSS STORIES

7. Adding positive Physical + Mental + Spiritual +Emotional investments are recipes and keys to a balanced diet.

8. You are not the reflection staring back at you in the mirror but the person standing there.

9. When breaking the cycle of poor eating habits, it's imperative to not only examine the now but explore what lead you to your present and plan for your future. Find or search for the influencers and not the ingredients.

10. No one has the perfect diet neither do you have to be flawless to get started.

11. Self-love minus determination to live a life that loves yourself, is equal to staying in the same place expecting different results.

12. Many lose weight in public and but it right back on in private. It is possible to put on weight and gain back simultaneously.

13. The thought we place on food should give you food for thought. Interview your food before you consume it. What is your food made up of? What is the background of your food? Does your food choice have any references or a proven track record of success?

14. Feed yourself Yes (your earthy substances) Food instead of eating No (nothing organic) food.

15. You are not what you ate last but a byproduct of what you will eat.

Dr. Oliver T. Reid "Your Solution Coach"
www.iamasolutionconsultingllc.com

YUMMY RECIPES

Rockin' Roasted Hummus

- Recipe by Inspirational Eve

Ingredients:

2 1/2 cups canned chickpeas (or 2 cans of BPA free chickpeas

2 tbsp. Tahini (you can also use creamy peanut butter)

6 tbsp. olive oil, divided

3 tbsp. warm water

1 large bulb of garlic

Juice from 1 fresh lemon

Salt and pepper to taste

Directions:

1. Preheat oven to 300 degrees. Cut off tops of garlic bulb so the majority of garlic cloves are slightly exposed.

2. Coat garlic bulb with 2 tbsp. of olive oil. Set the rest of the olive oil to the side. Wrap garlic bulb in foil and roast in the oven for 1 hour. Allow to cool.

3. Using fingers, squeeze cooled garlic out of their husks and into a food processor or blender.

4. Rinse and drain the chickpeas. Add chickpeas along with all other ingredients into the food processor or blender. Blend until completely smooth, about 4 minutes. You may need to scrap the sides and continue to blend.

The Besto Vegan Pesto

- Recipe by Inspirational Eve

Ingredients:

2 cups basil leaves

2 garlic cloves

1/2 cup nutritional yeast (or Parmesan if you want it non-vegan)

1/3 cup pine nuts (or almonds)

1/2 cup olive oil

Salt and Pepper

Directions:

1. Using a food processor or blender, process basil and garlic until finely chopped.

2. Add nutritional yeast and pine nuts. Pulse into a coarse paste.

3. With the machine on, slowly add the olive oil until incorporated. Season with salt and pepper.

4. Can be stored in the refrigerator for up to a week. Serve on pastas, vegetables, pizza or use a dip for vegetables.

Strawberry Salsa

- Recipe by Inspirational Eve

Ingredients:

2 cups strawberries, leaves removed and berries chopped

1 cup avocado, chopped

1/2 cucumber, chopped and seeded

2 tbsp honey or agave

1 tsp lime zest

2 tbsp juice from a lime (about 2 limes)

2 tbsp jalapeno, chopped optional

Salt and pepper to taste

Directions:

1. Pre-chop all ingredients. In a large bowl, mix all your ingredients together until full incorporated. Serve with bread or tortilla chips!

Meatless Monday Chili

- Recipe by Inspirational Eve

*Use BPA-free cans

Ingredients:

2-14oz cans kidney beans, drained

1 can pinto beans, drained

1 can black beans, drained

1 can no salt added tomatoes

1 block of vegetable bouillon mixed in 2 cups hot water

2 tbsp. olive oil

2 cups fresh or frozen corn.

1 small yellow onion, diced

2 garlic cloves, minced

2 bell peppers (red, yellow, orange preferably) diced

1 tbsp cumin

2 tbsp chili powder

2 tsp cinnamon

Morning Star meat crumbles, optional

Directions:

1. Drain and thoroughly rinse all your beans. Place all beans in a large bowl and set aside. Chop onions, garlic and peppers. Set aside.

2. In a large saucepan, heat olive oil over medium heat. Add corn and sauté for 4 minutes or until golden. Set corn aside.

3. In the same pan, add in onions and sauté until golden, about 5 minutes. Add in garlic and cook one more minute. Add in beans, tomatoes, broth and spices. Bring to a boil.

4. Once boiling, bring heat down to low and simmer for 10 minutes.

5. While chili is simmering, in a large sauce pan, sauté your package of meat crumbles according to package directions. Add into your chili.

6. Serve with sour cream and green onions.

ORGANIZED OBSTACLES: A COLLECTION OF WEIGHT LOSS STORIES

Breakfast Popsicle

- Original Recipe by The Frosted Vegan

Perfect for healthy quick summer breakfast on the run

Ingredients:

2 cups almond milk or other non-dairy milk

1 banana, frozen

1 tsp vanilla

1 tbsp. maple syrup

1/2 cup blueberries, fresh or frozen

1/3 cup granola, any variety preferably gluten-free

Directions:

1. Blend together almond milk, vanilla, maple syrup and banana in the bowl of a blender or food processor. 2. Fold or stir in granola and blueberries. I chose not to blend the granola and blueberries in in order to maintain the chunks of the goodness.

3. Pour into Popsicle molds, make sure not to overfill. Freeze for at least 2 hours.

4. Depending on your popsicle mold, you may need to run warm water over the mold for a few seconds until the popsicles easily slide out. Store in a sealed bag in the freezer for up to 2 weeks.

<u>*Taco Lasagna*</u>

- Recipe by Inspirational Eve

Makes 2 personal lasagnas

Ingredients:

1 cup green lentils

1 cup vegan beef bouillon

Olive oil

1/4 cup onion, sliced thinly

2 garlic cloves, minced

1/3 cup red cabbage, diced

1/4 cup bell pepper, diced

1/4 cup zucchini, cubed

Salt and Pepper

Vegan refried beans

6 corn tortillas

For Tomato Sauce

3 Roma tomatoes, diced

3 tbsp. tomato paste

1 tbsp. hot sauce

1/4 cup green or black olives, minced

Salt and Pepper

For Mango Salsa

1 mango, seeded and cubed

2 tbsp. onion, minced

1/2 jalapeno, minced

1 tbsp. fresh lemon juice

2 tbsp. bell pepper, chopped

Cilantro

Salt and Pepper

Directions:

1. Preheat oven to 350 degrees. Over high heat in a large saucepan, bring 2 cups of water to a boil. Add lentils and beef bouillon, and simmer on medium until lentils have absorbed the liquid, about 15 minutes.

2. Meanwhile, heat 2 tablespoons of olive oil in a large skillet over medium heat. Add onion, sauté for 3 minutes. Add garlic, cabbage, bell pepper, and zucchini, cooking 5 more minutes. Season with salt and pepper and set aside.

3. To make the tomato sauce, mix all the ingredients in a bowl until fully incorporated. Salt and pepper to taste and set aside.

4. Once lentils are cooked you can start to assemble to lasagna. Place one corn tortilla down on an oven safe plate. Spread an even layer of the refried beans on the tortilla. Top with a big scoop of lentils. Add another tortilla and top with onion and cabbage mixture. Add another tortilla, spread an even layer of refried beans and lentils then top with tomato sauce.

5. Repeat to make other lasagna and bake for 10 minutes.

6. To make salsa, mix all ingredients in a bowl and top each lasagna with it.

Healthy Peanut Butter Cups

- Recipe by Inspirational Eve

Ingredients:

2 cups dark chocolate chips

1/4 cup coconut oil

1 cup peanut butter or almond butter

2 tbsp. maple syrup

Directions:

1. In a double boiler or medium sauce pan, melt chocolate chips. Add in coconut oil and stir until fully incorporated.

2. Using mini cupcake liners, place all liners on a cookie sheet. Pour enough chocolate to cover the bottom of the mini cupcake liners. Set in the freezer for 10 minutes to set.

3. Meanwhile, mix peanut butter with maple syrup until incorporated.

4. Remove cups from freeze. Spoon a small amount of peanut butter in the middle of the cups. Pour the rest of the chocolate over top of the peanut butter to cover completely. Place in the freezer for 60 more minutes to set up.

BBQ Pulled Eggplant

- Recipe by Inspirational Eve

Ingredients:

1 eggplant

Olive Oil

1/4 cup onion, sliced thin

2 garlic cloves, minced

3/4 cup BBQ sauce

Directions:

1. Preheat oven to 375 degrees.

2. Wash and dry your eggplant. Slice eggplant in half lengthwise. Rub olive oil over eggplant and place on a greased baking sheet with eggplant cut side down in olive oil.

3. Bake for 45 minutes. Remove from oven and allow to cool for about 10-15 minutes

4. Meanwhile, heat olive oil in a large skillet over medium-high heat. Add onion and sauté for 5 minutes. Add in garlic and cook for 1 more minute.

5. Remove skin from eggplant and squeeze out the excess moisture.

6. Shred eggplant with your hands, removing flesh from the dark purple skin. Add to the skillet and sauté for 1 minute. Add BBQ sauce and cook 3 more minutes.

7. Serve on gluten-free buns or inside taco shells!

Cauliflower Buffalo Wings

- Recipe by Inspirational Eve

Ingredients:

1 large head of cauliflower

1 cup water

1/2 cup gluten-free flour

4 tbsp. vegan butter

1/2 cup Frank's Red Hot Sauce

Directions:

1. Preheat the oven to 300 degrees. Line a cookie sheet with parchment paper.

2. Rinse the cauliflower and let dry. Break the cauliflower into large florets. Set aside.

3. In a bowl, mix the water and flour together until combined.

4. Working in batches, dip each floret in the flour mixture then place on the cookie sheet. Continue with the rest of the florets. Bake for 15 minutes.

5. In a bowl, stir together the butter and hot sauce. Heat on the stove or in the microwave until butter is melted. Set aside.

6. Take 'wings' out of the oven, pour the hot sauce evenly over all the wings. Return back into the oven for 15 more minutes.

7. Let cool for 5 minutes.

Spicy Chickpea Bites

- Recipe by Inspirational Eve

Ingredients:

2 (15 ounce cans) organic chickpeas

2 tbsp. olive oil

1 tsp chili powder

1/2 tsp garlic powder

1/2 tsp cayenne pepper

1/2 tsp salt

Directions:

1. Preheat oven to 400 degrees. Drain and thoroughly rinse chickpeas in a strainer. Let drip dry.
2. Combine the chickpeas and all other ingredients in a large power, stirring until full incorporated.
3. Spray a large cookie sheet with nonstick spray. Add the chickpeas to the cookie sheet, spreading them out into an even layer.
4. Bake for 35 minutes or until crunchy.

Recipes submitted by Inspirational Eve
www.inspirationaleve.com

ORGANIZED OBSTACLES: A COLLECTION OF WEIGHT LOSS STORIES

ABOUT THE BOOK CREATOR

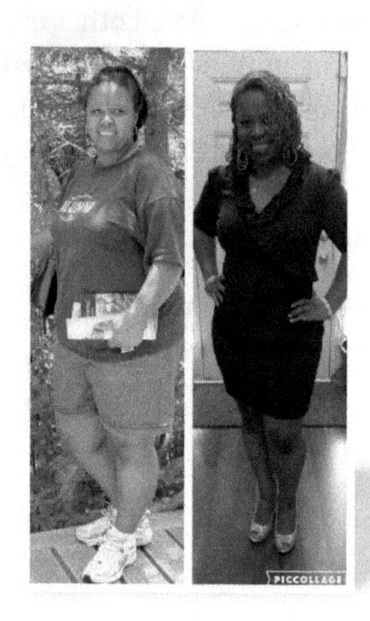

Some may know her as The Success Instigator but before that she was known as Blind, Broken and Bankrupt. To understand the woman, you must understand her "story":

At the age of 5 an accident left her BLIND in one eye....
At age 25 she was left BROKEN as a Single Mother....
At age 34 a loan scam left her to file BANKRUPTCY....

Despite these 3 B's...she became:
*Power Speaker
*Author Extraordinaire

ORGANIZED OBSTACLES: A COLLECTION OF WEIGHT LOSS STORIES

*And Success Instigator!

Rhonda uses her story and life lessons to instigate others how to P.U.S.H...Pursue Until Success Happens!

She is currently a Corporate Trainer and Author. More importantly she is not just another motivational speaker, she is a Success Instigator. Her ability and connection with audiences has featured her in several blogs, radio programs and even Essence Magazine. She lives in North Carolina with her teenage daughter.

ABOUT THE CONTRIBUTORS

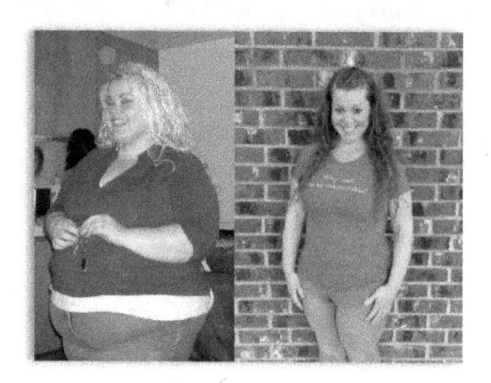

Inspirational Eve

Inspirational Eve is a nationally known life coach, body positive advocate and neuro-linguistic programmer. She has transformed her body, mind and spirit through self-love, self-care and the act of releasing the traumas from her past. Eve started her journey in 2010 as a 340 pound drug addicted woman with a self-sabotaging nature. From releasing 150 pounds and keeping it off since, she now helps other women release unsupportive behaviors from their minds, bodies and spirit. Eve lives in Denver, Colorado where she teaches Self-Love workshops along with weight release workshops, women's empowerment events and co-creator of the successful weight loss program the Discovery Diet.

For more information on Eve and how to start your weight release journey, visit www.inspirationaleve.com

ORGANIZED OBSTACLES: A COLLECTION OF WEIGHT LOSS STORIES

Melinda Squires

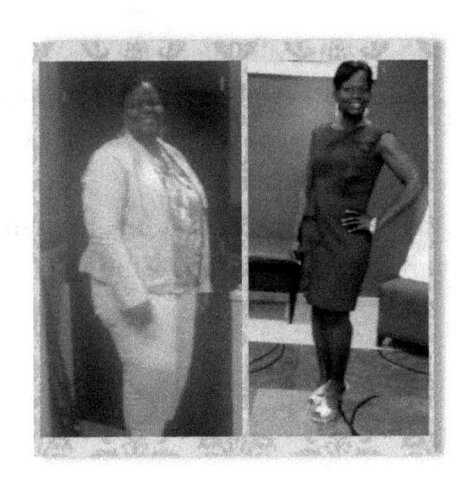

Melinda Squires was born on August 11, 1971 to the Late Billy Lee Midgette and Joanetta Squires on the East Coast of North Carolina, New Bern. She is the 2nd daughter of three children. She graduated from Pamlico County High School in June 1989 where she began course work towards a Bachelors of Business Administration at North Carolina Central University (NCCU) in Durham NC. She completed her studies at NCCU in May 1995. After graduation, she remained in the Raleigh-Durham and started her career at International Business Machines (IBM) as a Business Analyst, where she was employed for ten years before being laid off. She later gained employment with the City of Durham where she has served the Citizens of Durham for nearly fourteen years in several positions. Currently, she's a Senior Corporate Budget & Management Analyst with the City of Durham's

ORGANIZED OBSTACLES: A COLLECTION OF WEIGHT LOSS STORIES

Budget and Management Services Department. She is a single mother of a fourteen year old son, Darrius who is the love of her life. She's an active member of her Church, Peach Missionary Baptist Church. Her hobbies include: running, reading, braiding hair, traveling, and family gatherings and shopping.

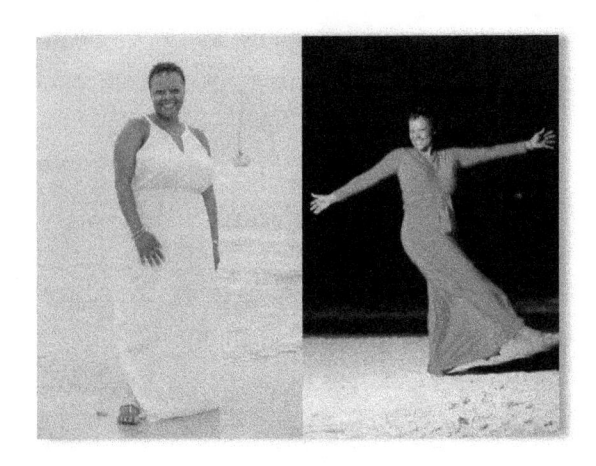

ORGANIZED OBSTACLES: A COLLECTION OF WEIGHT LOSS STORIES

Tina C. Hines

Tina C. Hines, is a compassionate and enigmatic certified life, empowerment, and transformational coach, who has devoted her life's works to inspiring, motivating and guiding women to leap into their dreams through live coaching in self-love, self-care and self-worth.

Tina began cultivating her expertise in coaching during her 30 year career in corporate America. She has managed executive offices at the Robert Wood Johnson Foundation, Black Enterprise Magazine and Johnson & Johnson.

Tina has lived an inspired life guided by the practice of meditation as well as journal writing. She has a firm belief that inner harmony transcends into outer beauty. She has gently walked the paths of inner peace gathering knowledge, rooting experience and reaping a myriad of

ORGANIZED OBSTACLES: A COLLECTION OF WEIGHT LOSS STORIES

benefits that she passes on to women so they too may blossom into full fruition through the realization of their self-worth.

Tina's unique spirit, stern commitment and distinctive method of pairing tough love with deep compassion which awakens her clients to embracing the self-love that will permit them to become more than they imagined possible, has gained her recognition as a lead expert in her field.

At present, Tina travels throughout the United States and Caribbean for private sessions, workshops and empowerment retreats, educating, empowering, and enlightening professional women. Her goal is simple. To encourage women to embrace who they are outside of being executives and mothers, alongside sharing her transformation techniques in meditation and journal writing.

Tina has been featured in the NY Times and on Good Morning America and was twice awarded 50 Fabulous Female Entrepreneurs and 101 Women You Should Connect With, Follow and Know on Social Media. Tina is one of the co-authors of Her Story HIS Glory, stories of women who have survived suicide and defeated depression. The book is scheduled for release the end of 2015 and will further Tina's work to empower and transform even more lives.

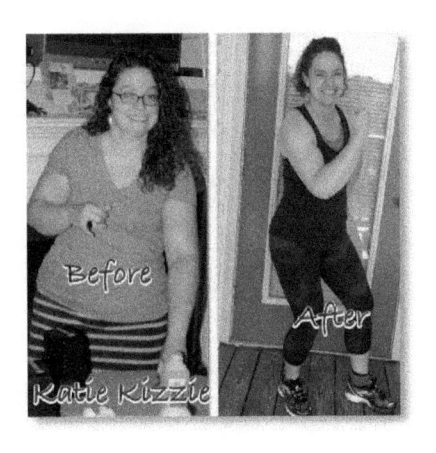

ORGANIZED OBSTACLES: A COLLECTION OF WEIGHT LOSS STORIES

Katie Kizzie

In 2014, I was a 34-year-old mother of two children who had never exercised consistently nor paid any attention to the foods that I was eating. No matter what weight, I saw myself as the chunky kid in my aunt's size 14 dress in my third grade fall picture. My heaviest weight came at 215 pounds during my first pregnancy. After my son, the scale started creeping up again and I was tired of hearing myself make excuses; I decided to make a change. Boot camp workouts and better nutrition have allowed me to be healthier and happier, positively impacting my entire family and myself!

ORGANIZED OBSTACLES: A COLLECTION OF WEIGHT LOSS STORIES

Icy Barzey-George

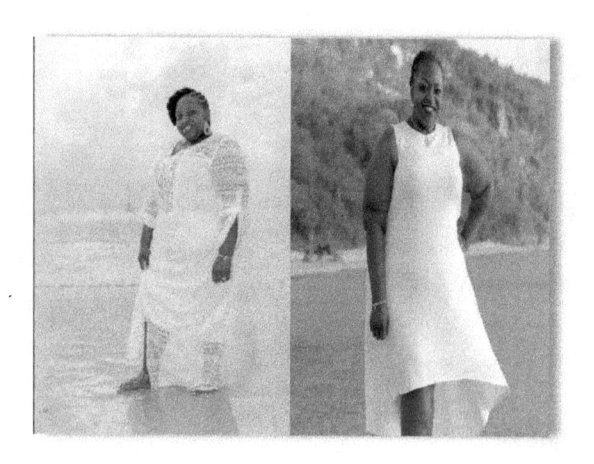

Icy Barzey-George is a wife and mother of 2, who is a loving, charismatic ball of energy that feels her life purpose is to uplift and pour love and positive enlightenment of self into every person she comes in contact to, because there was a time in her life, that she didn't think that she was worthy of that same love, until now!

Icy has worked in the geriatric sector as a Clinical Dietitian for the past 25 years, and came to the reality that it was time for a "rebirth."

Icy has added Total Life Changes to her coaching business and became an Independent Business Owner in the company, where she has recently excelled in sale and team building to be promoted to Executive

Director in Total Life Changes. For Icy, her weight journey has set off a series of events that allow her to share her story publically and inspire others via social media; as a result she is currently working on workshops for self-care and self-love through the art of meditation and affirmation writing.

Icy is currently finishing her studies in Life Coaching and is working on writing her first of many books to uplift, and inspire other to press the "rebirth" button. You can follow Icy on social media at:

www.Facebook.com/Theweightisovernow. You can visit www.GetFirWithIcy.Fit and learn about her health and wellness products. For nutrition counseling or inquiry about Total Life Changes health and wellness products, and her weight journey, Icy can be contacted at Icybgeorge@gmail.com or call 718-490-2043.

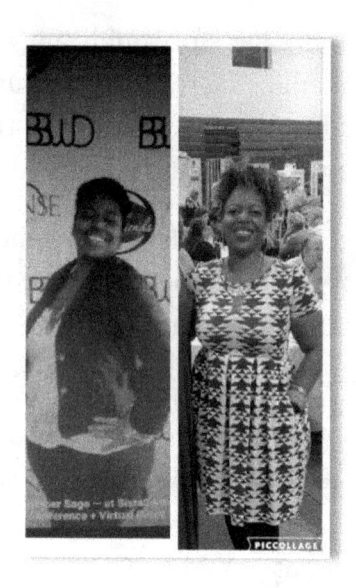

ORGANIZED OBSTACLES: A COLLECTION OF WEIGHT LOSS STORIES

Katrina Harrell

This story of how I released 100+ lbs. of physical weight is for the seen unseen, the heard unheard, the judged and the many who desperately cry out for validation from within but whose scars were visible and literally wreaking havoc on them, their purpose and destiny. Where the life they didn't choose is killing them swiftly and by their own hands. I stand and speak truth and life in death and lies and misconceptions about what it means to be obese. This isn't a story of losing physical weight, but of self-love and purpose and courage to love your scars – both seen and unseen – so that they may be healed.

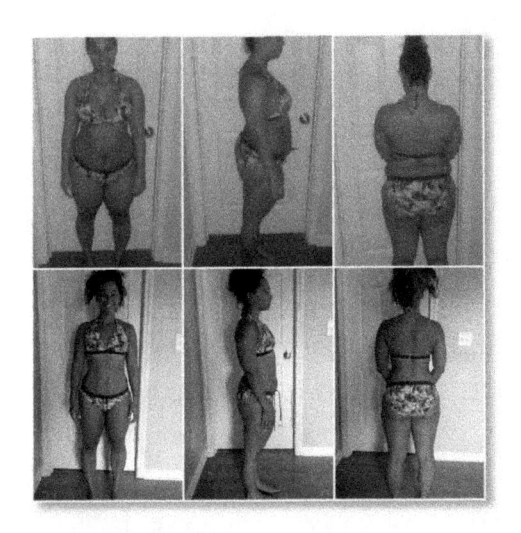

ORGANIZED OBSTACLES: A COLLECTION OF WEIGHT LOSS STORIES

Christin Pearson

Pregnancy...a beautiful and amazing experience, which does crazy things to our bodies. I was blessed to have two boys in 2 years, yes you read that correctly. They are 15 months apart. After being pregnant for two years and essentially taking 1.5-2 years off from my passion, I realized that getting "my body" back was not going to be the easiest thing I have done. I mean seriously, who has time to work out with 4, yes FOUR children. So here we are...LIFE HAPPENS, right?

This is the part where I had to **STOP** and say *"I am important too."* We live for our children, and we want to continue to live and be there for them each and every day...so we have to be healthy for ourselves but also for them, right? Right! Each day I dedicated 1-2 hours for ME, and ONLY Me! And what did I do? I exercised and

ORGANIZED OBSTACLES: A COLLECTION OF WEIGHT LOSS STORIES

exercised! SWEAT IS BEAUTIFUL!!! Sweat is the fat Crying!! I made lots and lots and lots of sweat daily!!! I also changed my eating tremendously, no more cravings, no more fatty foods. I changed my lifestyle, because I knew it would be something I would have to be able to do forever in order to keep a healthy lifestyle for myself....and my family!

I went from 180 pounds, 41% body fat, to 138 and 29% body fat in 6 months. Was this easy? NO, it most certainly was not the easiest thing I have done. Some days were hard, some days were easy. Did I ever have a cheat meal, cheat day, cheat week? YES, YES, and YES. It is important to cheat....NOT every day and certainly not every week, but I do understand that sometimes life gets the best of us, sometimes we are UNABLE TO get out of our own minds, and sometimes it is just HARD!!! After the 6 months did I continue on my lifestyle change? YES and it was easier than before. Some days are still hard, some days I still have cravings, some days I am weak and give in.

My mission is to simply to help any Lady of P² Fitness feel the same, to reach limits they NEVER thought would be possible, to reach for the stars and actually touch them.

Christin Pearson
Owner/Head Trainer of P² Fitness
www.Psquaredfitness.com

ORGANIZED OBSTACLES: A COLLECTION OF WEIGHT LOSS STORIES

ORGANIZED OBSTACLES: A COLLECTION OF WEIGHT LOSS STORIES

AUTHOR CREATOR INFORMATION:

Rhonda Nails

919-972-8510

www.rhondanails.com

ORGANIZED OBSTACLES: A COLLECTION OF WEIGHT LOSS STORIES

PUBLISHER/EDITOR:

Angel B. Inspired Inc.
P.O. Box 49647
Greensboro, NC 27419
(704) 978-8679
www.angelbarrino.com
www.angelbinspired.com
angelbinspired@gmail.com

Cover Art: Alegna Media Designs
www.alegnamediasuite.com

Interior Support: DH Bonner Virtual Solutions LLC
www.dhbonner.net

CPSIA information can be obtained
at www.ICGtesting.com
Printed in the USA
BVHW042134120423
662273BV00012B/396